BARIATRIC AIR FRYER COOKBOOK

100+ RECIPES FOR HEALTHIER FRIED FAVORITES THAT ARE EASY TO MAKE AND DELICIOUS TO EAT THAT WILL HELP YOU EAT WELL AND LOSE WEIGHT.

By: Bailey Caldwell

TABLE OF CONTENS

TABLE OF CONTENS 2

INTRODUCTIONS 4

    1. Breakfast Casserole 7
    2. Spinach Muffins 9
    3. Broccoli Muffins 11
    4. Zucchini Gratin 13
    5. Egg Bite 14
    6. Honey Nut Granola 16
    7. Vegetable Frittata 17
    8. Breakfast Potatoes 19
    9. AVOCADO TAQUITOS 20
    10. Mushroom, tomato and ham frittata 21
    11. Broccoli, Cheddar & Spinach Frittata 23
    12. Trout Frittata 25
    13. Potato Hash 26
    14. Turkey Burritos 27
    15. Bowl Baked Oatmeal 29
    16. Chicken Omelette 32
    17. Spicy Sweet Potato Hash 33
    18. Jalapeño Potato Hash 35
    19. Spinach and Eggs Scramble 36
    20. Veggie Quiche 37
    21 Shakshuka 39
    22. Indian-Style Cauliflower 42
    23. Prawn Pickle 43
    24. Zucchini Salad 44
    25. Breakfast Cobbler 45
    26. monkfish with olives and capers recipe 47
    27. butter and garlic baked 48
    28. Ranch Tilapia 50
    29. FRIED CRAB STICKS 51
    30. Banana Oatmeal 52
    31. Herb-Roasted Shrimp 53
    32. COCONUT SHRIMP 54
    33. Tuna-Stuffed Zucchini 57
    34. LEMON BAKED COD FISH 58
    35. GARLIC BUTTER HERB SCALLOPS 60
    36. Rabas 62

37. Salmon with Sweet-and-Sour Pan Sauce 63
38. Fried Catfish 64
39. Parmesan Crusted Tilapia 66
40. Homemade Fish Sticks 67
41. PASTA WITH SHRIMP, ZUCCHINI, & CHERRY TOMATOES 68
42. Honey Garlic Glazed Salmon 70
43. Crumbed Fish 71
44. salted salmon 73
45. Trout Almondine 74
46. Fish Nuggets 76
47. CREAMY GARLIC BUTTER SALMON 77
48. Baked Cod with Tomatoes and Onions 79
49. Steamed Mussels with Peppers 81
50. Cajun Salmon 83
51. Baked Salmon with Garlic and Dijon 84
52. Chili-Garlic Glazed Salmon 86
53. GARLIC BUTTER BAKED SALMON 87
54. Simple Garlic Shrimp 89
55. SPICY OVEN FRIED CATFISH 91
56. Halibut with Balsamic Glaze 93
57. Lemon Pepper Salmon 94
58. CRISPY TILAPIA 97
59. Crisp Fried Prawns 98
60. Prawns with garlic butter 100
61. GRILLED GARLIC SHRIMP WITH SAFFRON 101
62. Healthy Lemon Vegetable & Fish Foil Packets 102
63. Asian Salmon Foil-Pack Dinner 104
64. Chicken Broccoli Stir Fry 105
65. Chicken Fajitas 107
66. Chicken Hash 109
67. Chicken Nuggets 111
68. CHICKEN THIGHS 112
69. Chicken Parmesan 114
70. Pan-Roasted Chicken and Vegetables 116
71. Chicken Wings 117
72. Crumbed Chicken Tenderloins 119
73. General Tso's Chicken 120
74. Lemon Pepper Chicken 124
75. Keto Fried Chicken 126
76. AIR FRYER TURKEY BREAST 127
77. Keto Fried Chicken 129
78. Creamy Cajun Chicken 131

79. Chicken paprika 133
80. Korean Fried Chicken 134
81. Sweet and Sour Chicken 137
82. CHICKEN TIKKA MASALA 139
83. Herb-Roasted Turkey Breast 141
84. Maple Roast Turkey 143
85. Caribbean Chicken 145
86. Chicken Piccata 146
87. Thai Chicken 148
88. Spicy Dry-Rubbed Chicken Wings Recipe 149
89. Pecan Crusted chicken 151
90. Chicken Meatballs 154
91. EASY CHICKEN TACOS 156
92. Air Fryer Fried Chicken KFC Copycat 157
93. Oregano Chicken 160
94. Turkey Brine 161
95. Blackened Chicken 162
96. Thyme-Roasted Turkey Breast 164
97. Alfredo Chicken Wings 165
98. Chicken Drumsticks 167
99. Turkey Meatballs 168
100. Steak Salad 170
101. SESAME BEEF STIR FRY 172
102. BEEF FILLET STEAKS WITH PEPPER THYME SAUCE 174
103. Cranberry Meatballs 175
104. BEEF FILLET STEAKS WITH PEPPER THYME SAUCE 177
105. HONEY GARLIC PORK CHOPS 179
106. Ham with Orange-Apricot Sauce 181
107. Sausage, Peppers, and Onions 182
108. Chocolate Chip Cookie Recipe 184
109. Garlic and Rosemary Grilled Lamb Chops 186
110. Ham with Orange-Apricot Sauce 187

INTRODUCTIONS
BARIATRICS

What Does Bariatric Mean?

You've probably heard the word "bariatric," but what precisely does it imply?

A simple Google search reveals that bariatric refers to "relating to or specialized in the treatment of obesity." When you hear the term "bariatric" used in a medical context, it refers to obesity treatment, prevention, and causes.

Obesity is a dangerous health problem marked by excess body fat that can have a significant impact on your well-being. Type 2 diabetes, heart disease, high blood pressure, sleep apnea, osteoporosis, and stroke are just a few of the chronic diseases related to it.

Obesity is highly widespread in the United States; according to a survey done by the Centers for Disease Control and Prevention (CDC), over 40% of people in the United States were obese in 2015-16.

Whenever a person's body mass index (BMI) is equal to or more than 30, they are considered obese, they are categorized as obese and may be referred to as a bariatric patient. BMI is a formula for calculating weight in proportion to height.

Your BMI range determines which obesity category you fall into. Obesity is classified as Class 1 when the BMI is 30-34.9, Class 2 when the BMI is 35-39.9, and Class 3 when the BMI is 40 or more. Your chance of getting chronic illnesses increases as your BMI rises.

Bariatrics is a medical specialty that focuses on and treats obese people to help them lose weight and improve their overall health via food, exercise, and behavioral treatment. You might think of bariatric surgery, also known as metabolic or weight-loss surgery, when you think about bariatrics.

Weight-loss procedures, such as a roux-en-Y gastric bypass or a vertical sleeve gastrectomy, are used to help patients who are obese lose weight. Weight-loss surgery can also help to prevent or reverse the onset of chronic illnesses.

Although the word "bariatric" is commonly used, it does not automatically imply surgery.

Items designed specifically for obese people to meet their demands are referred to as bariatric. A bariatric scale, for example, is a scale designed specifically for those who are obese. Other bariatric gadgets are specially designed to give convenience and comfort to bariatric patients and can be used to move, help, and aid them.

RECIPE

1. BREAKFAST CASSEROLE

Prep Time: 10 minutes

Cook Time: 55 minutes

Total Time: 1 hour 5 minutes

Ingredients

- 2 pounds pork sausage
- 12 eggs
- 1 cups ofour cream (light or regular)
- 1/4 cup ofmilk
- salt and pepper
- 4 green onions
- 1/2 green bell pepper, diced
- 1/2 red bell pepper, diced
- 2 cups of shredded cheddar cheese

Instructions

Preheat the oven to 350 degrees Fahrenheit. Coat a 9x13-inch baking pan with making spray.

In a big mixing bowl, whisk together the eggs, sour cream, milk, cheese, and salt and pepper. Electric mixers should be used to blend the ingredients on low speed.

Over medium heat, heat a large skillet. Cook the sausage until it is browned, breaking it up with a wooden spoon as it cooks. Take the sausage from the casing and place it in the bowl with the egg mixture.

In same pan as the sausages, fry the potatoes, add the bell peppers and onion and cook for 2- 3 minutes. Stir everything together in the mixing bowl with the eggs.

Bake for 35-50 minutes, or until the sides are firm and the middle is just slightly jiggly, in a greased 9x13" pan.

Leftover egg casserole may be kept in the fridge for 3-4 days and eaten. Microwaving leftovers is a wonderful way to reheat them.

Nutrition

Calories: 385kcal | Carbohydrates: 2g | Protein: 23g | Fat: 30g | Saturated Fat: 12g | Cholesterol: 239mg | Sodium: 669mg | Potassium: 327mg | Sugar: 1g | Vitamin A: 705IU | Vitamin C: 11.6mg | Calcium: 194mg | Iron: 1.8mg

2. SPINACH MUFFINS

Prep Time: 10 minutes

Cook Time: 22 minutes

Total Time: 32 minutes

Ingredients

- 18 standard cupcake liners
- 2 cup offlour, whole wheat
- 1 1/2 tsp cinnamon
- 2 tsp baking powder
- 1/2 tsp baking soda
- 1/4 tsp salt
- 1/2 cup ofbutter, unsalted
- 3/4 cup ofmilk
- 1/2 cup ofhoney
- 1 large banana
- 6 ounce raw baby spinach (by weight)
- 1 large egg
- 1 tsp vanilla extract

Instructions

Warm the oven to 350° F and prepare a muffin tin with paper liners (or use silicone muffin cups of sprayed with cooking spray).

Joint all of the dry ingredients in a full of water basin.

Melt the butter in a saucepan over low heat. In a large mixing bowl, puree the raw spinach, banana, honey, milk, egg, vanilla, and melted butter until smooth.

Pour the puree into the dry ingredient dish and stir it in slowly until all of the ingredients are completely combined. (Be cautious not to over-mix the ingredients.)

After spooning the mixture into the muffin pan, cook for 18-22 minutes, or until the muffins are firm to the feel but not yet browned.

Allow it to cool for the most, if not all, of the time before serving.

Nutrition

139 calories, 20 grams of carbohydrates, 3 grams of protein, 6 grams of fat, 4 grams of saturated fat, 25 milligrams of cholesterol, 85 milligrams of sodium, 2 grams of fiber, and 9 grams of sugar.

3. BROCCOLI MUFFINS

Prep Time: 10 minutes

Cook Time: 20 minutes

Total Time: 30 minutes

Ingredients

- 2 heads broccoli to yield 2 cups ofbroccoli rice
- ¼ cup ofonion diced
- 1 cups ofharp cheddar cheese shredded
- 1 egg lightly beaten; large or extra large
- Salt and pepper as need optional; we used ⅛ tsp of each

Instructions

Preheat the oven to 350 degrees Fahrenheit.

Wash and thoroughly dry broccoli before making broccoli rice. Pull the florets off the stems. Cut the stalks into tiny pieces after peeling off the outer covering of flesh.Combine all of the items in a mixing bowl and pulse several times until the broccoli is finely chopped.

2 cups of broccoli rice 2 cups of broccoli rice 2 cups of broccoli rice 2 cups of broccoli rice 2 cups of broccoli rice 2 cups of broccoli Use any leftover broccoli rice for anything else.

In a big mixing bowl, mix 2 cups of broccoli rice, onion, cheddar cheese (and salt and pepper, if desired).

In a big mixing bowl, mix the broccoli and egg.

Scoop the mixture into micro or standard muffin pans that have been sprayed with nonstick cooking spray. About 24 tiny muffins or 8-9 normal sized muffins will be produced. Overfilling the muffin tray is ok since the mixture settles as it cooks. You may, however, receive less than the quantity stated.

Using the back of a spoon or your fingers, press the mixture down.

Cook for 20 minutes, or until firm and browning begins.

Remove from tins gently and enjoy!

Nutrition

Calories: 24kcal | Protein: 1g | Fat: 1g | Saturated Fat: 1g | Cholesterol: 11mg | Sodium: 34mg | Potassium: 33mg.

4. ZUCCHINI GRATIN

Prep: 10 min

Cook: 55 min

Ingredients

- 6 tbsp (3/4 stick) unsalted butter, + extra for topping
- 1 pound yellow onions, cut in 1/2 and sliced (3 large)
- 2 pounds zucchini, sliced 1/4-inch thick (4 zucchini)
- 2 tsp kosher salt
- 1 tsp freshly ground black pepper
- 1/4 tsp ground nutmeg
- 2 tbsp all-purpose flour
- 1 cup of hot milk
- 3/4 cup of fresh bread crumbs
- 3/4 cup of grated Gruyere

Directions

Preheat oven to 400 degrees Fahrenheit.

In a very large (12-inch) saute pan, melt the butter and sauté the onions for 20 minutes, or until soft but not browned. Cook, covered, for 10 minutes or until zucchini is soft. Cook for another 5 minutes, uncovered, with the salt, pepper, and nutmeg. Add the flour and mix well. Cook for a few minute over low heat, until the heated milk has thickened into a sauce. Fill an 8-by-10-inch baking dish halfway with the mixture.

Toss the bread crumbs and Gruyere together and sprinkle over the zucchini mixture. Bake for 20 minutes, or until bubbling and golden, with 1 tbspof butter chopped into tiny pieces.

5. EGG BITE

Prep Time 3 minutes

Cook Time 10 minutes

Ingredients

- 4 large eggs
- 2 Tbs. cottage cheese
- 2 Tbs. shredded cheese
- 1/8 tsp. salt and pepper

Red Pepper and Bacon Mix Ins

- 3 slices bacon cooked and diced
- 1 Tsp. roasted red peppers, chopped

Tomato Feta Mix Ins

- 1/4 cup oftomatoes, diced
- 1/4 cup offeta cheese

Mexican Mix Ins

- 1/4 cup oftomato, diced
- 1/4 cup ofonions, diced
- 1/4 cup ofbell peppers, diced

- 1 T. salsa

Veggie Mix Ins

- 1/8 cups ofpinach, chopped
- 1/8 cup ofonion, diced
- 1/8 cup ofmushrooms
- 1/8 cup ofbell peppers, diced

Instructions

mix eggs, shredded cheese, salt & pepper, and cottage cheese in a small mixing bowl. mix.

Connect the egg bit maker.

Fill a cup ofhalfway with water and pour it onto the heating plate's bottom.

Use a non-stick spray to coat silicone molds.

Fill the bottoms of the cups of with mix-ins. The ingredients for the mix-ins are given above. To avoid overflowing, pour the egg mixture over the mix-ins, filling them about 3/4 full.

Cook for 7-10 minutes, or until all of the liquid has evaporated.

Turn the cups of over and discard the egg pieces.

Sour cream, chives, bacon, pico, and other toppings work well with your mix-ins.

Disconnect the plug from your egg bite maker.

6. HONEY NUT GRANOLA

Prep:10 mins

Cook:20 mins

Total:30 mins

Ingredients

- 4 cups of rolled oats
- 1 cups ofliced almonds
- 1 cup ofchopped pecans
- 1 cup ofraw sunflower seeds
- ⅓ cup ofcanola oil
- ½ cup ofhoney
- 1 tsp vanilla extract
- 1 tbspground cinnamon

Instructions

Warm the oven to 300 degree Fahrenheit (150 degrees C).

mix the oats, almonds, and sunflower kernels in a large mixing basin. mix the oil, honey, vanilla, and cinnamon in a separate bowl. Mix thoroughly with the dry ingredients. Spread the mixture onto two baking sheets that haven't been greased.

Bake for 10 minutes in a preheated oven, then remove and stir.Return to the oven for another 10 minute, before golden brown. Remove the baking sheet from the oven and cool completely before storing it.

Nutrition

Per Serving: 188 calories; protein 3.7g; carbohydrates 19.9g; fat 11.1g; sodium 1.4mg. Full Nutritio

7. VEGETABLE FRITTATA

PREP TIME:10 mins

COOK TIME:15 mins

TOTAL TIME:25 mins

INGREDIENTS

- 6 eggs
- 1/4 cup offull fat yogurt optional
- 1 cups ofhredded mozzarella cheese divided
- ¼ cup ofred onions chopped
- 1 cup ofmushrooms chopped
- 8-10 stalks asparagus ends trimmed and chopped
- ¼ cup ofcilantro chopped
- ½ cup ofcherry tomatoes sliced

INSTRUCTIONS

Preheat oven to 425 degrees Fahrenheit.

mix the egg, yogurt, half of the shredded mozzarella cheese, and salt and pepper in a mixing bowl; leave aside.

In an oven-safe or cast iron pan, heat the olive oil. Cook for 3-5 minutes, until the onions, mushrooms, and asparagus are softened.

On top of the cooked veggies, pour the egg mixture. Add the remaining cheese and the cut cherry tomatoes on top.

Bake uncovered in a preheated oven for 10-15 minutes, or until the middle is firm and not jiggly.

NOTES

Leftovers should be stored in a closed bag.They'll keep in the fridge for up to three days.
Instructions for Freezing: The frittata may be stored in the freezer for up to three months. Warm by defrosting overnight in the refrigerator and baking brfore well cooked at 350°F. However, I would avoid reheating in the microwave since it may cause the veggies to lose too much moisture and have a rubbery texture.
Substitutes: For the best results, stick to the original recipe. However, several popular alternatives that might work well in this recipe are listed below.

Yogurt is purely a personal preference. For a richer texture, add ricotta or sour cream instead of yogurt. Regular milk or plant-based milk can also be used.

You can use any other veggies in place of the ones listed.

You may use any type of cheese instead of the cheddar.

NUTRITION

Calories: 216kcal, Carbohydrates: 6g, Protein: 17g, Fat: 13g, Saturated Fat: 6g, Cholesterol: 271mg, Sodium: 288mg, Potassium: 355mg, Fiber: 1g, Sugar: 3g, Vitamin A: 975IU, Vitamin C: 7.6mg, Calcium: 223mg, Iron: 2.2mg.

8. BREAKFAST POTATOES

Prep Time: 10 mins

Cook Time: 35 mins

Ingredients

- 1 pound small potatoes, cut into ½-inch pieces
- Extra-virgin olive oil, for drizzling
- ½ tsp smoked paprika
- Pinch of red pepper flakes
- Sea salt and freshly ground black pepper

Optional sautéed onions & peppers

- ½ tsp extra-virgin olive oil
- ½ yellow onion, chopped into ½-inch pieces
- 1 red pepper, chopped into ½-inch pieces
- 2 garlic cloves, chopped
- ⅓ cup ofcilantro, for serving
- Sea salt and freshly ground black pepper

Instructions

Warm the oven to 425°F and place parchment paper on a baking pan. Place the potatoes on the baking sheet, drizzle with olive oil, and season with salt, pepper, smoked paprika, and red pepper flakes as need. Toss to coat, then spread out evenly on the baking sheet and bake for 30 minutes, or until golden brown and crunchy around the edges. Stop here and serve plain or with onions and peppers sautéed in butter.

To make the onions and peppers, start by chopping them up. In a medium skillet, heat the oil over medium heat. Sauté the onions, peppers, and garlic for 5 to 8 minutes, or until soft and lightly browned. Take the pan from the warm, add the potatoes, and top with cilantro.Season to taste with salt and pepper, and serve right away.

9. AVOCADO TAQUITOS

Prep Time:5 minutes

Cook Time:6 minutes

Total Time:11 minutes

Ingredients

- 6-8 corn tortillas
- 2-3 medium avocados
- 3/4 cup ofMexican blend cheese
- salt and pepper as need

Instructions

In a fry pan, warm the oil over medium heat.

In a bowl, mix the avocados, cheese, salt, and pepper. Fill each corn tortilla with about a quarter cup ofthe filling. Wrap it up and drop it into the oil seam-side down.

Cook till golden brown on both sides. Allow excess oil to drop off on a paper towel-lined plate.

Nutrition

Calories 244Calories from Fat 117% Daily Value*Fat 13g20%

Saturated Fat 7g44%,Cholesterol 42mg14%,Sodium 326mg14%

Potassium 110mg3%,Carbohydrates 18g6%,Fiber 2g8%

Protein 12g24%,Vitamin A 290IU6%,Calcium 324mg32%

Iron 0.7mg4%

10. MUSHROOM, TOMATO AND HAM FRITTATA

PREPARATION TIME:10 Mins

COOK TIME:20 Mins

INGREDIENTS:

- 4 eggs
- 2 cherry tomatoes
- 6 button mushrooms
- 1 slice smoked ham
- 2 tbspcheddar cheese
- Salt and pepper
- 1 tbspbutter

Instructions

Lightly mix the eggs in a big mixing basin.

Season with salt and pepper then add cherry tomatoes, mushrooms, ham, and cheese.

In a small saucepan, melt the butter (use one that is oven-proof). Fill the pan halfway with the egg mixture and cook over medium heat until the edges are slightly hard.

To make big curds, use a fork to pull the egg from the edges to the center.

Reduce the warm to low and cook for another 3–4 minute.

Cook for another 5 minutes in a preheated oven at 180 degrees Celsius, or until the top is golden brown.

Cut the frittata into ornamental shapes using a cutter or slice it into squares with a knife.

Serve with chives as a garnish.

11. BROCCOLI, CHEDDAR & SPINACH FRITTATA

Prep Time: 15 mins

Cook Time: 25 mins

Total Time: 40 minutes

INGREDIENTS

- 8 SimplyNature Organic Cage Free Eggs
- ½ cup ofmilk of choice
- 2 small-to-medium cloves garlic, pressed or minced
- ½ tsp sea salt, divided
- Freshly ground black pepper
- 1 cup offreshly grated cheddar cheese, divided
- 1 tbspSimplyNature Organic Extra Virgin Olive Oil, more as needed
- 1 small yellow onion, chopped
- ⅓ cup ofwater
- 2 cups of thinly sliced broccoli florets
- 2 cups of SimplyNature Organic Baby Spinach, roughly chopped
- ⅓ cup ofthinly sliced green onions

INSTRUCTIONS

Preheat the oven to 425 degrees Fahrenheit. Whisk together the eggs, milk, garlic, 14 tsp salt, and approximately 5 twists of freshly ground black pepper in a big mixing bowl before thoroughly mixd. Then whisk in half of the cheese, keeping the other half for another time.

Heat the olive oil in a 10-inch cast iron skillet or oven-safe sauté pan over medium heat until it shimmers. mix the onion and the remaining 14 tsp salt in a mixing bowl. Cook, turning often, for 3 to 5 minutes, or until the onion is soft and transparent.

Add broccoli and water in the pan, cover with a lid (or a baking sheet), and steam for 2 to 3 minutes, or before the broccoli is brighter green and easily penetrated with a fork. Take the lid and stir in the spinach and green onions. Cook, stirring frequently, for 30 to 60 seconds, or until the spinach has wilted.

Spread the mixture evenly on the pan with a spatula.Finally, whisk the egg mixture and pour it into the pan. The remaining cheese should be sprinkled over the frittata. Bake until you can shimmy the pan by the handle (careful, it's hot!) 12 to 15 minutes later, check to see whether the centre is just just set.

Allow 5 to 10 minutes for the frittata to cool before slicing it into 6 big or 8 smaller wedges. Serve right away. Leftover frittata can keep for up to 3 days if covered and refrigerated. Serve cold or reheated gradually.

NOTES

ELIMINATE THE DAIRY: Omit the cheese and use a neutral-flavored, unsweetened non-dairy milk.

CHANGE IT UP: Simply omit the spinach for a traditional broccoli-cheddar frittata. Alternatively, use your favorite greens—baby arugula and chard would be delicious.

12. TROUT FRITTATA

Total: 25 min

Active: 25 min

Ingredients

- 8 large eggs, at room temperature
- 1/2 cup of heavy cream, at room temperature
- 3 tbsp extra-virgin olive oil
- 1 bulb fennel, chopped fine
- 1 shallot, chopped fine
- 1/2 tsp kosher salt
- 10 cherry tomatoes, halved
- One 4-ounce fillet smoked trout, flaked, skin and bones removed
- 1/4 cup of fresh basil leaves, torn
- 2 ounces fresh goat cheese

Directions

Preheat the broiler to its highest setting.

Mix the eggs and cream together in a medium mixing bowl until fully smooth. Eliminate from the equation.

Over medium-high heat, heat an oven-safe 10-inch skillet. Heat for a few seconds after adding the oil. Add the fennel and shallots and simmer for 3 minutes, or until the fennel has softened. Add salt and pepper, then add the tomatoes and fish and continue to cook for another minute. Simmer for 1 minute, stirring regularly, after pouring the egg mixture over the fish. Scrape the bottom of the pan lightly with a rubber spatula to bring up some of the cooked egg. Rep 3 times more. Spread the mixture evenly in the pan (the top will still be liquid) and top with basil and goat cheese.

3 to 4 minutes under the broiler, until the frittata is cooked through and lightly browned on top. Allow it cool for a few minute before slicing and serving.

13. POTATO HASH

Total: 35 min

Active: 35 min

Ingredients

- 1 russet potato, scrubbed
- 1 sweet potato, scrubbed
- 3 tbsp salted butter
- 1 cup ofchopped red bell peppers
- 1 cup ofchopped yellow squash
- 1 cup ofchopped zucchini
- 1/2 red onion, chopped
- Salt and freshly ground black pepper
- 4 large eggs

Directions

Pierce each potatoes many times, place in the microwave, and heat on high for 5 to 10 minutes, or until cooked through. Remove the sweet potato's peel with care. Set aside the diced potatoes.

2 tbsp butter, melted in a medium pan over medium heat Cook for a few minutes after adding the bell peppers, squash, zucchini, and onions. Cook until the diced potatoes are golden brown, then add them to the vegetables. Salt & pepper as need.

Melt the remaining tbspof butter in a separate pan over medium heat and crack in the eggs. Cook for 3 to 4 minute, or before the whites have set.

Serve each serving of hash with a fried egg on top.

14. TURKEY BURRITOS

Prep:5 mins

Cook:20 mins

Total:25 mins

Ingredients

- 1 pound ground turkey
- 2 (7.75 ounce) cans Mexican-style hot tomato sauce (such as El Pato®)
- 1 whole kernel corn (15.25 oz.) can, drained

- ½ small onion, diced
- 1 (16 ounce) can fat-free refried beans
- 1 (16 ounce) container fat-free sour cream
- ¾ cups ofhredded reduced-fat Cheddar cheese
- 6 (10 inch) flour tortillas

Instructions

Brown ground turkey in a big pan over medium-high heat. mix tomato sauce, corn, and onion in a mixing bowl. Reduce the warm to medium-low and continue to cook, stirring periodically, until the liquids have reduced (about 20 minutes).

Warm the beans in a separate medium pan over medium-low heat. Toss the sour cream and cheese into the burritos before serving. Warm tortillas one at a time over a stove flame for 1 to 2 minutes, turning once or twice. Beans come first, followed by the meat combination, sour cream, then cheese. Fold the top over and serve while it's still hot.

Nutrition

Per Serving: 571 calories; protein 33.8g; carbohydrates 78.4g; fat 7.9g; cholesterol 75.9mg; sodium 1549.1mg. Full Nutrition

15. BOWL BAKED OATMEAL

Prep Time: 5 minutes

Cook Time: 35 minutes

Ingredients

- 1 and 3/4 cups of (420ml) milk (dairy or nondairy)
- 2 large eggs*
- 1/2 cup of(120ml) pure maple syrup*
- 1/4 cup of(60g) unsalted butter, melted and slightly cooled
- 1/4 cup of(60g) unsweetened applesauce or mashed banana
- 3 cups of (240g) old-fashioned whole oats
- 1 tsp baking powder
- 1 tsp ground cinnamon
- 1 tsp pure vanilla extract
- 1/4 tsp salt
- 1 and 1/2 bowl of mixed berries, fresh or frozen (do not thaw)
- optional for topping: 1/2 cup ofchopped walnuts or pecans

Instructions

Warm the oven to 350 degrees Fahrenheit (177 degrees Celsius) and set the oven rack in the bottom third position. Using nonstick spray, coat a 9-inch or 11-inch baking pan. Any pan of similar size or shape will do, however an 8-inch pan will be too tiny. For a 913 inch pan, see the recipe note.

In a large mixing basin, mix all of the ingredients. Pour onto the baking pan that has been prepared. If desired, garnish with nuts. (Alternatively, mix into the oatmeal.) Bake for 35 minute, or before the center is almost set, resulting in a soft oatmeal like the one seen above. Bake until the center has set for drier, more firm baked oats.

Allow 5 minutes to cool before serving. If preferred, spoon or slice and serve with yogurt. Refrigerate leftovers securely covered for up to 1 week.

Notes

Make Ahead Instructions: Bake the oats, let it cool fully, then keep it in the refrigerator for quick breakfasts throughout the week. Reheat in the microwave or bake for 10 minutes at 350°F (177°C) in a 350°F (177°C) oven. Bake and chill oatmeal before freezing. Freeze for up to 3 months if firmly wrapped. Thaw at room temperature or in the refrigerator. Warm to your preference. I like to divide the cooled baked oats into bars or portions and freeze them separately for a quick breakfast. Place each in a big freezer bag or container, wrapped with plastic wrap.

Make sure you don't make the oatmeal batter ahead of time. All of the liquid will be absorbed by the oats! mix all of the ingredients in a mixing bowl, then bake right immediately. For an alternative, see the make-ahead directions above.

Eggs connect the casserole and give it a delicious taste. If necessary, you can substitute 1/3 cup ofunsweetened applesauce or mashed banana for the eggs.

Sugar: I prefer using pure maple syrup since it has a fantastic taste and keeps the baked oats extra moist! You can also use honey, coconut sugar, or packed brown sugar.

What a lovely flavor of butter! Without it, the baked oatmeal can taste rubbery. Replace with a fat-free substitute. Melted coconut oil is a great dairy-free alternative.

Oats: The finest texture comes from whole oats. Quick oats absorb more moisture, causing the baked oatmeal to dry out. If you're using steel-cut oats, soak them in milk for 20 minutes before adding the rest of the ingredients. Increase the baking time for a few minute.

Add-ins: Use the same quantity of peeled chopped apples, peaches, pears, bananas, or other fruit instead of berries. 1 cup ofchocolate chips, dried cranberries, nuts, or raisins, or 1 cup ofchocolate chips, dried cranberries, nuts, or raisins

913 inch Pan: To make a 913 inch pan, double the recipe. The baked oats will be extremely thick and will need to bake for at least 10 minutes longer. If the edges are browning too rapidly, cover them with aluminum foil.

Nutrition

Calorie 227, Total Fat 8g, Carbohydrate 34g, Dietary Fiber 4g, Sugars 15g, Protein 5g.

16. CHICKEN OMELETTE

Prep Time 5 minutes

Cook Time 8 minutes

Ingredients

- 4 eggs
- 1 tbsp coconut oil (or use another oil such as olive oil)
- 1/3 cup ofcut, cooked chicken
- 3 tbsp tomato, chopped
- 3 tbsp shredded mozzarella cheese
- handful fresh spinach
- sea salt
- ground black pepper

Instructions

Mix the eggs together in a little bowl until they are smooth.

Add the coconut oil to a big pan on the stove over low heat. Pour the eggs into the pan after the coconut oil has melted. Season the eggs with salt and pepper, and cook for a few minutes, or until the edges begin to brown.

Cook for a few minute more after adding the chicken, cheese, tomato, and spinach to half of the omelette.

Cook for a few more minutes, before golden and cooked through, folding the omelette in half with a spatula.

Notes

Feel free to substitute another oil, such as olive oil, for the coconut oil. Simply leave out the cheese to make this omelette dairy-free. For this omelette, you may use whatever cheese you like.

You can add whatever veggies you love to this omelette.

Nutrition

Calories 274Calories from Fat 19% Daily Value*,Fat 22g34%

Saturated Fat 12g75%,Cholesterol 352mg117%,Sodium 271mg12%,Potassium 174mg5%,Carbohydrates 2g1%,Fiber 1g4%,Sugar 1g1%,Protein 18g36%,Vitamin A 810IU16%,Vitamin C 3mg4%,Calcium 161mg16%,Iron 2mg11%

17. SPICY SWEET POTATO HASH

Prep:10 mins

Cook:15 mins

Total:25 mins

Ingredients

- 2 strips uncured chicken bacon
- 2 medium sweet potatoes, cubed
- 1 tbspolive oil, or more as needed
- 1 large jalapeno pepper, finely choppe
- 1 ½ tbsp BBQ sauce

- 1 tsp garlic powder
- 1 pinch ground dried chipotle pepper
- salt and ground black pepper as need

Instructions

Cook the bacon in a big pan over medium-high heat, stirring periodically, for approximately 5 minutes, or until uniformly browned. When cool enough to handle, drain on paper towels and crumble.

Microwave the cubed sweet potatoes in a microwave-safe bowl on high power for 5 minutes while the bacon cooks.

Over medium heat, heat a large skillet. Add the sweet potatoes, garlic powder, chipotle powder, salt, and black pepper once the olive oil has been added. Cook for 5 to 7 minute, or before potatoes are golden and crisp. Cook for another 2 to 3 minutes over low heat with the bacon, jalapeño, and BBQ sauce.

Note:

If you're using normal potatoes, microwave them for up to 8 minutes and cover your skillet to achieve uniform browning.

Nutrition

279calories; protein 3.9g; carbohydrates 51.3g; fat 7g; sodium 256.5mg.

18. JALAPEÑO POTATO HASH

Prep time :3mins

Cook time: 12mins

INGREDIENTS

- 1 1/2 tablespoons extra-virgin olive oil (distributed)
- 1 medium golden potato, diced
- 1/ 4 yellow onion, chopped
- 1/ 2 jalapeno pepper, finely chopped
- 1/ 4 avocado, sliced
- 1 egg
- 1 tsp parsley, freshly chopped
- Parmesan cheese, for sprinkling
- Crushed red pepper, As need

INSTRUCTIONS

1 tbspolive oil, heated in a large cast-iron pan over medium heat. Cover and cook potatoes, onions, and jalapeo for 7-8 minutes, stirring often. Place in a serving dish or on a serving plate.

In a separate, small pan, heat the remaining 1/2 tbspolive oil over medium-low heat. Cook for 3-4 minute, before the whites are set and the yolk is still runny, by cracking one egg immediately into the pan. Arrange the potatoes on top of the egg. As need, top with avocado, parsley, parmesan, and red pepper.

19. SPINACH AND EGGS SCRAMBLE

Prep Time: 10 mins

Cook Time: 10 mins

Total Time: 20 mins

INGREDIENTS

- 2 tbsp olive oil
- ½ medium onion, sliced and separated into rings
- ½ tsp Diamond Crystal kosher salt + a pinch for the onions
- ¼ tsp black pepper, divided
- 4 large eggs
- 2 tbsp grated Parmesan (1 oz)
- 2 cups of fresh baby spinach leaves (2 oz)
- ¼ tsp red pepper flakes

INSTRUCTIONS

2 minutes over medium-high heat, heat a very big (12-14 inch) nonstick skillet. Pour in the olive oil.

Place the onion pieces on top. Using a sprinkle of Kosher salt and a pinch of black pepper, season them. Cook, stirring periodically, for approximately 5 minutes, or until golden. Reduce the heat to a medium setting.

Combine the eggs in a medium mixing basin, 12 tsp Kosher salt, a sprinkle of black pepper, and 2 tbsp Parmesan while the onion is frying. Eliminate from the equation.

Add the spinach leaves to the pan when the onions are golden brown. Cook, stirring constantly, for approximately 1 minute, or until the spinach begins to wilt.

Fill the skillet with the egg mixture. Cook the eggs over medium warm, moving them around with a rubber spatula until they are set to your taste. Red pepper flakes may be used as a finishing touch. Serve right away.

NUTRITION

Serving: 0.5recipe | Calories: 303kcal | Carbohydrates: 4g | Protein: 16g | Fat: 25g | Saturated Fat: 6g | Sodium: 612mg | Fiber: 1g | Sugar: 2g

20. VEGGIE QUICHE

Prep Time:20 minutes

Cook Time:40 minutes

Total Time:1 hour

Ingredients

- avocado oil, 1 tsp (or whatever type of oil you prefer)
- 1/2 onion, thinly sliced
- 1 seeded red pepper, cut into thin strips
- 1 tsp. garlic, minced
- 1/2 pound chopped mushrooms
- 2 bowl of loosely packed spinach

- 1 refrigerated pie crust
- 1 1/2 cups of milk (I used whole milk but 2% is fine)
- 5 eggs
- 1/4 tsp. salt
- 1/4 tsp. pepper
- 8 tsp. nutmeg
- 1/2 cup ofgrated cheese (sharp cheddar, swiss, or gruyere work great)

Instructions

Preheat the oven to 350 degrees Fahrenheit.

In a medium-sized pan, heat the oil. Sauté the onions and peppers for 2-3 minutes, or until the onions begin to become transparent.

Cook, stirring occasionally, before the mushrooms are cooked through, about 5 minutes. Cook for one additional minute, or before the spinach has wilted. Pull the pan off the heat and set it aside.

Refrigerated pie dough should be unrolled and pressed into a 9-inch pie pan. Eliminate from the equation.

Whisk the eggs until they are foamy. Whisk together the milk, salt, pepper, and nutmeg.

Using a kitchen towel or paper towels over the sink, squeeze the cooked veggies to remove any excess liquid (this keeps the crust from getting soggy).

Arrange the vegetables in an equal layer on top of the dough in the pie pan. Cheese should be sprinkled on top. In an even layer, pour the egg mixture over the veggies and cheese.

Bake for 40-45 minutes, before the top begins to brown. Take from the oven and set aside to cool for 5-10 minutes before slicing and serving.

Nutrition

Calories: 287kcal | Carbohydrates: 21g | Protein: 12g | Fat: 17g | Saturated Fat: 6g | Cholesterol: 152mg | Sodium: 343mg | Potassium: 399mg | Fiber: 1g | Sugar: 5g | Vitamin A: 1950IU | Vitamin C: 29.9mg | Calcium: 175mg | Iron: 2mg

21 SHAKSHUKA

Prep Time: 15 minutes

Cook Time: 20 minutes

Total Time: 35 minutes

INGREDIENTS

- 2 tbsp extra virgin olive oil
- 1 sliced big yellow onion
- 1 big red bell pepper, diced (or 1 roasted red bell pepper)
- ¼ tsp fine sea salt
- 3 cloves garlic, pressed or minced
- 2 tbsp tomato paste
- 1 tsp ground cumin
- ½ tsp smoked paprika

- ¼ tsp red pepper flakes, reduce or omit if sensitive to spice
- a big can of crushed tomatoes (28 ounces), ideally cooked on an open fire
- 2 tbsp fresh cilantro or flat-leaf parsley, chopped, + addition cilantro or parsley leaves for garnish
- Freshly ground black pepper, as need
- 5 to 6 large eggs
- ½ cup ofcrumbled feta
- Crusty bread or pita, for serving

INSTRUCTIONS

Warm the oven to 375 degrees Fahrenheit (190 degrees Celsius). In a large oven-safe skillet (ideally stainless steel), heat the oil over medium heat. Add the onion, bell pepper, and salt once the pan is shimmering. Cook, stirring often, for 4 to 6 minute, before the onions are soft and transparent.

mix the garlic, tomato paste, cumin, paprika, and red pepper flakes in a large mixing bowl. Cook, stirring frequently, for 1 to 2 minute, before aromatic.

Add the cilantro and the smashed tomatoes with their juices. Stir the ingredients and bring it to a low simmer. Reduce the heat if needed to keep the sauce at a soft simmer, and cook for 5 minutes to let the flavors to mingle.

Turn the heat off. Taste (be cautious; it's spicy) and season with salt and pepper as needed. Make a well towards the perimeter with the back of a spoon and crack the egg immediately into it. To help contain the egg, pour a small amount of the tomato mixture over the whites. Depending on how many eggs you may fit, repeat with the remaining 4 to 5 eggs. Using a sprinkle of salt and pepper, season the eggs.

Transfer the pan to the oven with care (it's heavy) and bake for 8 to 12 minutes, checking frequently after the first 8 minutes. Whenever the yolk have dramatically risen and the egg whites are an opaque white but are still soft, they're done. When you shimmy the pan, they should still jiggle in the middle. (Remember that they'll continue to cook after you take the dish from the oven.)

Transfer the heated skillet to a heat-safe surface, such as the stove, using oven mitts (both hands!). If preferred, top with crumbled feta, fresh cilantro leaves, and more red pepper flakes. Serve in bowls with toasted bread on the side.

NOTES

OMIT THE FETA TO MAKE IT DAIRY-FREE. Top the shakshuka with halved and pitted Kalamata olives to compensate the saltiness.

TO MAKE IT VEGAN, FOLLOW THESE INSTRUCTIONS: While untraditional, I believe chickpeas (1 can, washed and drained, or 12 cups of cooked chickpeas) mixed in with the smashed tomatoes would be delicious. Eliminate the feta cheese from the recipe. Top the shakshuka with halved and pitted Kalamata olives to compensate the saltiness.

MAKE IT GLUTEN-FREE: The shakshuka is gluten-free in and of itself. If you don't want to eat gluten, use gluten-free bread.

NUTRITION

Vitamin A20%Vitamin C52%Calcium12%Iron19%Vitamin D11%Magnesium10%Potassium12%Zinc14%Phosphorus16%Thiamin (B1)14%Riboflavin (B2)34%Niacin (B3)13%Vitamin B628%Folic Acid (B9)15%Vitamin B1227%Vitamin E18%Vitamin K13%

22. INDIAN-STYLE CAULIFLOWER

PREP TIME:10 MINUTES

TOTAL TIME:25 MINUTES

Ingredients

- 2tbsp olive oil
- 1tsp coriander seeds
- 1tsp cumin seeds
- 1tsp curry powder
- 1tsp turmeric powder
- 1large head cauliflower, cored, broken into 1-inch florets
- Kosher salt and freshly ground black pepper
- 1easpoon finely grated peeled ginger
- 1tsp finely grated lime zest

INSTRUCTIONS

Preheat the oven to 450 degrees Fahrenheit. Combine the oil, coriander seeds, cumin seeds, curry, and turmeric in a large mixing basin. Season the cauliflower with salt and pepper. Toss to evenly coat the cauliflower. Arrange on a big rimmed baking sheet in a single layer (scrape any extra seasoning from bowl over cauliflower). Roast for 10–15 minutes, or until cauliflower is crisp-tender and golden around the edges. Place on a serving platter and top with ginger and lime zest. Warm or at room temperature is OK.

23. PRAWN PICKLE

Prep Time: 10 mins

Cook Time: 1 hr

Total Cook Time: 1 hr 10 mins

Ingredients

- 1/2 kg prawns, deshelled and deveined (pull out the vein)
- 1 cup ofcoconut vinegar
- 200 gm ginger
- 200 gm garlic
- 100 gm chilli powder
- 250 ml sesame oil
- Salt as need
- 2 tsp fenugreek (methi) seeds

Description

1.Refrigerate the prawns for 1 hour after marinating them with salt, 2 tsp chili powder, and two spoons of vinegar.

2.Roast the fenugreek (methi) seeds in the oven, then grind them and set aside. Take the vinegar from the heat and set it aside.

3.Warm the oil in a big pan with a thick bottom. Deep-fry the prawns but don't overcook them.

4.Add the ginger, sliced into long thin strips, to the same oil.

5. Saute for a few minute, then add the garlic and cook for another 2 minutes. Turn off the warm and stir in the chilli powder till the mixture is cool.

6. mix the fried prawns, salt, and vinegar in a mixing bowl and set aside to cool.

7. Keep in airtight glass bottles.

24. ZUCCHINI SALAD

Prep Time: 10 mins

Ingredients

- Lemon Vinaigrette, + 1/4 cup ofminced shallot mixed in
- 3 small-medium zucchini
- 1/4 cup oftoasted pine nuts
- 1 tbspchopped chives
- Handful of basil
- Shaved Parmesan, optional
- Sea salt and freshly ground black pepper

Instructions

Using a vegetable peeler, thinly slice the zucchini. Toss the zucchini with drizzles of the dressing in a large mixing basin, then transfer to a plate.

If using, garnish with pine nuts, chives, basil, and a few shavings of Parmesan. As needed, season with salt and pepper, then sprinkle with more dressing.

25. BREAKFAST COBBLER

Cook:45 mins

Prep:10 mins

Total:55 mins

Ingredients

- 5 cups strawberries, leaves removed and quartered, or enough to make a hearty layer on the bottom of your baking vessel (You can use whatever fruit you like here.) Really.)
- 1 tbsplemon juice (or about half a juicy lemon's worth)
- Cinnamon (as need, I like a lot)
- Brown sugar (as need, but probably around 2 tbsp)

Ingredients for the topping

- 1 cup ofwhite sugar
- 1 cup offlour
- 1/2 tsp salt (Maldon salt gives a nice crunch)
- 1 egg, lightly beaten
- 6 tbsp unsalted butter, melted (browned butter would be amazing here, too), + more for prepping the baking dish

Instructions

Warm the oven to 375 degrees Fahrenheit and grease an oven-safe baking dish. (Now is the ideal moment to utilize your cast iron pan.) A square, 10.5-inch cast iron skillet worked well for my companion and me.)

Pour the fruit into the prepared baking bowl, along with the lemon juice, cinnamon, and brown sugar. (If you don't want to use another bowl, combine all of the ingredients in the baking dish.)

To make the topping, whisk together flour, sugar, and salt, then add the lightly beaten egg. mix all of the ingredients before they are crumbly, then put on top of the fruit.

Over the topping, drizzle the melted butter.

Warm the oven to 350°F and bake the cobbler for 45 minutes, or until golden brown and bubbling.

Eat! (However, let it to cool for a few minutes.)

26. MONKFISH WITH OLIVES AND CAPERS RECIPE

Preparation Time: 10 mins

Cooking Time: 20 mins

Ingredients

- 4 monkfish fillets, 175g
- 1 slice of lime (zest and juice of)
- 1 peeled and finely chopped garlic clove
- 1 tablespoon extra virgin olive oil
- 1 pinch dried red pepper flakes + more for sprinkling
- 1 pinch Freshly ground black pepper
- 4 tbsp Low-fat natural yoghurt
- 25 g Pitted black olives, roughly chopped
- 1 tbsp Capers, rinsed and chopped
- 2 tbsp Fresh parsley, chopped
- 4 Lime wedges, to serve

Description

Warm the oven to 190°C/375°F/Gas mark 5 (190°C/375°F/Gas mark 5).

Strip any white membrane from the meat of the monkfish to prepare it. Sprinkle with lime zest and juice, garlic, olive oil, dried chili flakes (red pepper flakes), and black pepper in a roasting tin. Cook for 20 minutes, before the fish is well done.

Meanwhile, mix the yoghurt, olives, capers, and parsley in a mixing bowl and season as need with freshly ground black pepper.

Serve the fish with a huge green salad and lime wedges on the side, with the dressing on the side and a few dried chilli flakes (red pepper flakes) sprinkled on top.

27. BUTTER AND GARLIC BAKED SCALLOPS

Prep Time: 5 Minutes

Cook Time: 18 Minutes

Total Time: 23 minutes

INGREDIENTS

- 12 Medium scallops (clean and dry)
- 2 tbsp salted butter
- The juice of half a lemon
- Salt (as need)
- Pepper (as need)
- Garlic powder (as need)
- Sweet paprika (as need)

INSTRUCTIONS

Preheat the oven to 425 degrees Fahrenheit.

In an oven-safe casserole dish, equally distribute the clean scallops.

Squeeze the lemon juice over the scallops in an equal layer.

Using a sprinkle of salt, pepper, garlic powder, and paprika, season the scallops (as need).

Distribute the butter pieces equally around the scallops.

Baked Scallops with Butter and Garlic I LisaGCooks.com

Bake the scallops for 9 minutes before flipping them.

If necessary, season the scallops with salt, pepper, garlic powder, and paprika.

Return the scallops to the oven and bake for another 9 minutes.

Serve with fresh bread right away.

NOTES

You will know it is done when the center of the scallop will opaque and slightly hot.

On the scallops, I just squeezed lemon juice once.

Feel free as need and adjust the seasoning to your liking.

28. RANCH TILAPIA

Prep:15 Min

Cook:20 Min

Ingredients

- 6-8 tilapia fillets
- 1 pkg dry ranch dressing
- 1/2 c mayo
- 1 c plain bread crumbs
- 1/2 c parmesan cheese
- cooking spray {butter flavor}

Description

mix mayonnaise and dry Ranch dressing packet.
Place the bread crumbs and Parmesan cheese on a paper plate and set it aside.
Cover both sides of the fish with the herb mayo using a BBQ brush (I find this easiest if the fish is still slightly frozen).

Place each piece of fish on a prepared cookie sheet and dredge in the bread crumbs/cheese mixture. Smoothly spray the top of the fish with butter scented spray before baking for added crispiness.

Bake at 375°F for 8-12 minutes if partially frozen or 20-25 minutes if completely cold

Tips:

Fish that "flakes with a fork" is generally overdone and can be dry. This is an excellent test: Gently push on the cooked meat with your finger. The fibers will split into solid flakes when it's finished. The fish has been cooked too long

if the fibers fall apart.

29. FRIED CRAB STICKS

READY IN: 14mins

INGREDIENTS

- 8imitation crab sticks
- 3eggs
- 2tbsp milk
- 1 1/2 cups of panko breadcrumbs
- 1cup ofall-purpose flour
- vegetable oil (for deep frying)

DIRECTIONS

Preheat the vegetable oil to 350 degrees Fahrenheit. Take the crabsticks from their packaging and place them on foil or a platter. To make egg wash, whisk together eggs and milk.

One at a time, dredge each crab stick in flour. (Evevly coat.) The crabstick should next be dredged in egg wash. (Apply the mixture). After that, roll the crabstick in the panko breadcrumbs until it is thoroughly coated.

Steps 4–6 should be repeated for another two or three crabsticks.

Deep fried for about 2 minutes at 350 degrees, flipping once. (Be careful not to overcook the crab flesh, as it may separate into strips.)

Prepare the remaining crabsticks while these are cooking.

30. BANANA OATMEAL

Total Time: 10 minutes

Ingredients

- 1/2 cup of rolled oats
- 1/4 tsp salt
- 1 cup of milk of choice
- 1/4 cup of water or additional milk of choice
- 1 large very overripe banana, mashed
- optional 1/4 tsp cinnamon
- optional crushed walnuts, mini chocolate chips, shredded coconut, etc.
- sweetener of choice, if needed

Instructions

In a little saucepan, mix all of the ingredients. Over medium heat, bring to a boil. To avoid sticking or boiling over, just stir occasionally once the water has reached a boil. It will thicken with time. Sweeten as need. Toss in your preferred garnishes.

Peanut butter, micro chocolate chips, or the healthy nutella recipe mentioned previously in this piece are some of my favorites. Serve immediately, or chill overnight and serve hot or cold the next day.

31. HERB-ROASTED SHRIMP

Total: 30 mins

Ingredients

- 1 ½ pounds fresh or frozen jumbo shrimp (14 to 16 per lb.), thawed if frozen, peeled, and deveined
- 2 tbsp olive oil
- 2 tsp lemon juice
- 2 cloves garlic, minced
- 1 tsp salt
- 1 tsp chopped fresh marjoram or oregano
- 1 tsp chopped fresh thyme leaves
- Fresh Succotash Relish (optional)

Instructions

Preheat the oven to 375 degrees Fahrenheit. Dry the shrimp with a paper towel. In a 15x10-inch baking pan, arrange in a single layer. Drizzle the olive oil and lemon juice over the top. Garlic, marjoram, thyme, and 1 tsp salt are sprinkled over top. Roast for 8 to 10 minutes, uncovered, or until shrimp are opaque. This recipe serves 8 appetizers. Serve with Fresh Succotash Relish if preferred.

Nutrition

Per Serving: 94 calories; total fat 4g; saturated fat 1g; polyunsaturated fat 0g; monounsaturated fat 3g; cholesterol 119mg; sodium 379mg; potassium 201mg; carbohydrates 0g; fiber 0g; sugar 0g; protein 15g; trans fatty acid 0g; vitamin a 8IU; vitamin c 1mg; thiamin 0mg; riboflavin 0mg; niacin equivalents 0mg; vitamin b6 0mg; folate 0mcg; vitamin b12 0mcg; calcium 50mg; iron 0mg.

32. COCONUT SHRIMP

PREP:15 MINS

COOK:15 MINS

FREEZE:30 MINS

TOTAL:30 MINS

INGREDIENTS

- 1 pound (500 g) jumbo shrimp peeled and deveined, tails intact
- Salt and pepper
- 1/2 cup of all-purpose flour (plain flour)

BATTER:

- 1/2 cup of all-purpose flour (plain flour)
- 1 tsp baking powder
- 1/2 tsp garlic powder

- 1 egg
- 1/2 cup of beer (substitute with mineral water or soda water -- you may need a little extra)

COATING:

- 1 cups of hredded coconut sweetened or unsweetened
- 1 cup of Panko bread crumbs

INSTRUCTIONS

Using parchment paper, line a big baking sheet. Eliminate from the equation.

OPTIONAL: Insert a knife approximately three-quarters of the way through the top of the shrimp to butterfly it. Make a slit from the rear of the shrimp to the tail. To slightly open the shrimp flesh, use your fingertip. They don't have to be perfectly flat. Set aside after seasoning with salt and pepper.

Add 1/2 cup of flour to a shallow bowl for dredging. In a separate shallow basin, mix together the batter ingredients until smooth. The consistency of the better should be similar to that of pancake better. Thin the sauce with a bit more beer or mineral water if it's too thick, stirring after each addition.

Combine shredded coconut and bread crumbs in the third bowl.

Dredge in flour (shaking off excess), then dip in batter (shaking off excess), and last coat in breadcrumb/coconut mixture. Add a little coating of coconut on the shrimp.

Repeat with the remaining shrimp on the prepared baking sheet. Freeze the shrimp in a single layer until firm (about 30-45 minutes).

Heat vegetable oil (approximately 2-3 inches deep in the pot) in a dutch oven or deep pan until it is nice and hot.

FROZEN shrimp should be fried in batches for about 2-3 minutes each side, or until golden brown and crispy. Drain them on a paper towel-lined tray.

Serve with sweet chili sauce right away.

NOTES

Frying frozen shrimp prevents them from overcooking and allows the crumb to develop into that wonderful golden color. The coating is more durable and does not flake off.

You may still fry them as soon as you've finished breading them if you don't have time to freeze them. Just bear in mind that after a minute of heating, the crumb may start to come apart.

NUTRITION

Calorie: 417kcal | Carbohydrates: 46g | Protein: 30g | Fat: 11g | Saturated Fat: 7g | Cholesterol: 326mg | Sodium: 767mg | Potassium: 345mg | Fiber: 2g | Sugar: 10g | Vitamin A: 60IU | Vitamin C: 4.6mg | Calcium: 245mg | Iron: 5.3mg

33. TUNA-STUFFED ZUCCHINI

Prep:25 mins

Cook:25 mins

Total:50 mins

Ingredients

- 3 zucchini, trimmed ends
- 4 cans (3 oz.) tuna, drained and flakes
- ¼ onion, grated
- 1 tomato, finely chopped (Optional)
- 1 bowl of dry bread crumbs
- 1 egg, beaten
- salt and ground black pepper as need
- 1 tbspolive oil

Instructions

Fill a big saucepan halfway with salted water, add the zucchini, and cook for 5 minutes over medium heat to soften. Remove the zucchini from the pan, cut it in half lengthwise, and set it aside to cool.

Warm the oven to 350 degrees Fahrenheit (175 degrees C). Grease a 9x13-inch baking dish lightly. Scoop out the flesh and leave a 1/2-inch shell on the zucchini halves. In a bowl, set aside the meat that was scooped out. In a mixing basin, mash the zucchini flesh well. mix the tuna, onion, tomato, bread crumbs, egg, salt, and pepper in a mixing bowl. Fill the zucchini shells lightly with the tuna mixture. Drizzle roughly 1/2 tsp of olive oil over each zucchini half that has been filled. Cook for 20 to 25 minutes in a preheated oven until the tops are lightly browned.

Nutrition

Per Serving: 193 calories; protein 19.4g; carbohydrates 18.2g; fat 4.7g; cholesterol 48mg; sodium 209.1mg. Full Nutrition

34. LEMON BAKED COD FISH

Prep Time:5 MINUTES

Cook Time:10 MINUTES

Total Time:15 MINUTES

INGREDIENTS

- 4 portions cod fish
- 1/2 tsp salt
- 1/4 tsp black pepper
- 1/4 cups ofoftened butter
- 2 tbsp freshly grated parmesan cheese
- 1 tbspall-purpose flour
- 3 cloves garlic minced
- 1 tsp dried basil
- 1/2 tsp onion powder
- 1 tsp dijon mustard
- 1 lemon juiced

INSTRUCTIONS

Warm the oven to 400°F and oil a 9x13 baking dish lightly. Place the cod filets in the baking dish that has been prepared. Mix the fish with salt and pepper before serving.

mix the butter, parmesan, flour, garlic, basil, onion powder, dijon mustard, and lemon juice in a small mixing bowl.

A big spoonful of the butter mixture should be placed on top of each fillet.

Bake for about 10 minutes in a preheated oven. The thickness of your fish will affect the amount of time it takes to cook. It's done when the fish flakes readily with a fork.

Nutrition

Calories: 600kcal | Carbohydrates: 5g | Protein: 162g | Fat: 6g | Saturated Fat: 1g | Cholesterol: 389mg | Sodium: 830mg | Potassium: 3763mg | Vitamin A: 380IU | Vitamin C: 24mg | Calcium: 188mg | Iron: 3.9mg

35. GARLIC BUTTER HERB SCALLOPS

PREP TIME:10 MINUTES

COOK TIME:10 MINUTES

TOTAL TIME:20 MINUTES

Ingredients

- ⅓ cup ofkosher salt + more for seasoning1 cup ofhot water
- 1 Pound Large Scallops
- Salt and Pepper
- 1 Tbspolive oil
- 3 Tbsp butter
- 3 garlic cloves minced
- 1 tsp cup offreshly chopped oregano
- 1 tsp fresh rosemary chopped
- 1 teaspoon chopped
- fresh thyme, lemon wedges, and chopped parsley, if desired

Instructions

mix the salt and 1 cup ofhot water in a medium-sized mixing basin, stirring to dissolve the salt. To chill the brine, add ice water. Allow 10 minutes for the scallops to soak in the brine.A sheet pan lined with paper towels should be set aside.

Drain the scallops, rinse them under cold water, and place them in a single layer on a sheet pan lined with paper towels. Place second paper towel on top of the scallops and lighty wipe them down. To get the greatest browning results during cooking, remove as much surface moisture as possible.

In a medium pan, warm the oil over medium-high heat before it begins to smoke. Season the capers with salt and pepper before adding them to the skillet. Scallops should be seared for 3- 3 12 minutes on each side, or until golden brown. Take the pan and place on a plate to cool.

 mix the butter, garlic, and fresh herbs in a mixing bowl. Come back the scallops to the pan and cook for another 1-2 minutes to finish cooking. Serve with a piece of lemon and a sprig of fresh parsley on top.

36. RABAS

Preparation time 10mins

Cooking time 13mins

INGREDIENTS

- 1 Squid
- 1 Egg
- Flour
- Olive oil
- Salt
- 1/2 Lemon (optional)

Instructions

Squid should be cleaned and sliced into strips or rings.

Toss the squid with flour in a mixing basin.

In a separate container, beat the egg and season it with salt.

In a deep fry pan, warm the oil (the oil should be heated to 180 Celsius degrees or 365 Fahrenheit degrees).

Place the squid strips in the flour, then in the egg, and last in the pan.

To enhance the taste, serve with half a lemon (optional).

37. SALMON WITH SWEET-AND-SOUR PAN SAUCE

Ingredients

- 1 tbspvegetable oil
- ¼ cup offat-free, less-sodium chicken broth
- 2 tbsp brown sugar
- 2 tbsp fresh lime juice
- 1 tbsplow-sodium soy sauce
- 1 tbspfish sauce
- 2 garlic cloves, minced
- 4 salmon fillets (6 oz) (about 1 inch thick)
- ¼ tsp salt
- ¼ tsp freshly ground black pepper

Instructions

In a big nonstick skillet, warm the oil over low heat.
 mix the broth and the following five ingredients in a mixing bowl (broth through garlic).
Raise the warm to medium-high and cook for 3 minutes.
Season the fillets with salt and pepper as the pan warms up. Combine the fillets to the pan and cook for 4 minute on each side, or until the salmon flakes easily with a fork. Pull the fillets out of the pan. Samples were removed the fat from the pan. Scrape browned pieces from the bottom of the pan and add broth mixture. Bring to boil, then reduce warm to low and cook for 30 seconds. Remove the pan from the heat. Place the sauce on top of the fish and serve.

Nutrition

Per Serving: 309 calories; calories from fat 41%; fat 14.2g; saturated fat 3.3g; mono fat 5.9g; poly fat 3.8g; protein 37g; carbohydrates 6.3g; fiber 0.1g; cholesterol 87mg; iron 0.9mg; sodium 736mg; calcium 31mg.

38. FRIED CATFISH

PREP TIME:15 mins

COOK TIME:15 mins

TOTAL TIME:30 mins

Ingredients

- 4 to 6 catfish fillets (about 1-2 lbs.)
- 1 bowl ofmilk or buttermilk
- Salt
- 3/4 cup offine cornmeal (do not use coarsely ground cornmeal)
- 1/2 cup offlour
- 1 tsp garlic powder
- 1 tsp black pepper
- 1 tsp paprika
- 1/2 tsp cayenne
- 1/4 tsp celery seed
- For frying, oil (use peanut oil if you can)

Instructions

Heat the oil in the pan and the warming oven:

Pour enough oil into a sturdy frying pan (I use cast iron) to come 1/2 inch up the edges of the pan. On medium-high, heat the pan. Warm the oven to 200 degrees Fahrenheit and place a cookie sheet inside. On top of the cookie sheet, place a wire rack. Soak catfish in buttermilk or milk: Soak the catfish in milk or buttermilk while the oil heats up.

For dredging, mix cornmeal, flour, and spices:

Beat the cornmeal, flour, and spices in a mixing bowl. (Alternatively, you can use your preferred spice.) To dredge, place in a shallow dish. Dredge the fillets in flour, then cook them in heated oil: Allow the oil to reach 350°F; a simple test is to drop a little amount of dry breading into the oil and see whether it sizzles immediately.

Once the oil is warm, season the catfish fillets with salt and dredge them in the breading. Take off any excess and carefully place into the hot oil..Fry till golden brown, around 2-4 minutes, depending on the thickness of the fillet.Turn the salmon over with a metal spatula and cook for another 2-4 minutes.

Cast iron warms up quickly and stays hot, so keep an eye on the temperature while you fry; you may need to reduce the burner's heat at some time.

Warm fried fillets in the oven:

Place the fish in the oven once it's done cooking while you finish the rest of the catfish. The crispy texture of the fried catfish may be maintained by keeping it warm in the oven.

Serve immediately with your favorite spicy sauce, cole slaw, and hush puppies after they're all done.

39. PARMESAN CRUSTED TILAPIA

Prep Time: 5 mins

Cook Time: 12 mins

Total Time: 17 minutes

Ingredients

- 3/4 cup offreshly grated Parmesan cheese
- 2 tsp paprika
- 1 tbspchopped parsley
- 1/4 tsp salt (optional)
- 1 tbspextra virgin olive oil
- 4 tilapia filets (about 4 oz each)*
- lemon, cut into wedges

Instructions

Preheat the oven to 400 degrees Fahrenheit. Using foil, line a baking pan.

mix the Parmesan, paprika, parsley, and salt in a small basin. Drizzle the olive oil over the fish, then dredge it in the cheese mixture, softly pushing it in with your fingers if needed. Place the baking sheet on top of it.

Bake for 10-12 minutes, or until the thickest portion of the fish is opaque. Serve with lemon slices on the side.

Nutrition

Serving Size: 1 piece of fishCalories: 214Sugar: 0 gSodium: 505 mgFat: 12 gSaturated Fat: 5 gUnsaturated Fat: 5 gTrans Fat: 0 gCarbohydrates: 1 gFiber: 0 gProtein: 27 gCholesterol: 57 g.

40. HOMEMADE FISH STICKS

Total Time: 25 min

Ingredients

- 1/2 cup ofdry bread crumbs
- 1/2 tsp salt
- 1/2 tsp paprika
- 1/2 tsp lemon-pepper seasoning
- 1/2 cup ofall-purpose flour
- 1 large egg, beaten
- 3/4 pound cod fillets, cut into 1-inch strips
- Butter-flavored cooking spray

Directions

Warm the oven to 400 degrees Fahrenheit. mix bread crumbs and spices in a small bowl. Separate the flour and the egg in small basins. Coating both sides of the fish with flour and brush off excess.Dip in the egg, then in the crumb mixture, pressing it down to help the coating stick.

Spritz with butter-flavored cooking spray and place on a baking sheet covered with cooking spray. Bake 10-12 minutes, rotating once, or until salmon just begins to flake easily with a fork.

Nutrition

1 serving: 278 calorie, 4g fat (1g saturated fat), 129mg cholesterol, 718mg sodium, 25g carbohydrate (2g sugars, 1g fiber), 33g protein. Diabetic Exchanges: 4 lean meat, 1-1/2 starch.

41. PASTA WITH SHRIMP, ZUCCHINI, & CHERRY TOMATOES

prep time: 15 MINUTES

cook time: 20 MINUTES

total time: 35 MINUTES

INGREDIENTS

- 1/3 Cup ofExtra Virgin Olive Oil
- 4 Small Zucchini, Cut Into Coins
- 2 Cloves Garlic, Peeled & Sliced
- 1 Pint Cherry Tomatoes, Cut In Half
- 1 Pound Medium Shrimp, Peeled & Deveined
- 12 Fresh Basil Leaves, Thinly Sliced
- Pinch Red Pepper Flakes (Optional)
- Salt & Black Pepper

- 1 Pound Pasta

INSTRUCTIONS

In a big pan over medium warm, heat the oil, then cook the zucchini rounds on both sides until nicely browned.

Remove the zucchini with a scoop to a bowl and set aside.

For making the pasta, bring a big pot of lightly salted water to a boil.

Make the pasta according to the package directions before it is "al dente."

While the pasta is making, add the garlic to the pan in which the zucchini was made and simmer for a minute or two until fragrant over medium heat.

Cook for 3 to 4 minutes after adding the tomatoes to the garlic, then add the shrimp.

Cook, turning often, before the shrimp are pink and cooked through, about 5 minutes over medium heat.

To reheat, add the zucchini and cook for another 1 to 2 minutes.

Keep warm by adding the basil, salt, pepper, and pepper flakes if using.

Return the pasta to the saucepan after draining it and saving a small cup of the pasta water.

Toss the spaghetti with the shrimp mixture and make for a minute or two over high heat, until it is boiling hot, adding a little pasta water if required.

Represent with a sprinkling of parsley, minced.

42. HONEY GARLIC GLAZED SALMON

Prep Time: 8 minutes

Cook Time: 10 minutes

Total Time: 18 minutes

Ingredients

- 4 (6 oz each) salmon filets
- 1/2 tsp kosher salt
- 1/2 tsp black pepper
- 1/2 tsp smoked paprika
- 1/4 tsp blackening seasoning (optional)

SAUCE

- 3 Tbsp butter
- 2 tsp olive oil
- 6 cloves garlic minced
- 1/2 cup of honey
- 3 Tbsp water
- 3 Tbsp soy sauce
- 1 Tbsp sriracha sauce
- 2 Tbsp lemon juice

Instructions

Period the salmon with salt, pepper, paprika, and blackening spice after patting it dry (if using). Eliminate from the equation. Preheat the broiler after adjusting the oven rack to the middle position.

In a big oven-safe skillet, melt butter and oil over MED-HIGH heat. After the cheese has melted, add the onion, water, soy sauce, sriracha, honey, and lemon juice, and cook for 30 seconds, or until the sauce is heated through.

Cook for 3 minutes with the skin side down (if using skinned salmon). While the salmon is cooking, baste it periodically with the pan sauce by spooning it over the top.

Broil salmon for 5-6 minutes, basting once with sauce throughout the broiling process, or until desired doneness is reached.

43. CRUMBED FISH

Prep: 5 mins

Cook: 7 mins

Total: 12 mins

Ingredients

- 2 firm white fish fillets , skin off, at room temperature
- 2 tbsp dijon mustard
- Olive oil spray
- Salt and pepper

CRUMB

- 1/2 cup ofpanko breadcrumbs1 tbsp parsley , finely chopped

- 1/3 cup of(30g) parmesan , finely grated
- 1 garlic clove , minced
- 1 tbsp olive oil
- Pinch of salt

Instructions

Warm the grill or broiler to high heat.

To make the Crumbs, mix all of the ingredients in a mixing bowl and stir well to incorporate.

Season the fish on both sides with salt and pepper, then put mustard on top of each fillet (top only).

The mustard-smeared side of the fish should be pressed into the crumb mixture. To make it stick, press down hard. Then, for additional golden crumb, spritz with oil.

In a skillet, drizzle 1/2 tbspoil and cook over high heat.

Place the fillets in the heated skillet, then place on the grill / broiler (approximately 5"/15cm from the heat source) for 5 - 6 minutes, turning as needed, until the crumb is brown and the fish is cooked. Once cooked, the fish should flake in the middle.

Option 1: bake for 10-12 minutes at 220C/390F in the oven, then finish under the grill/broiler on high to get the crumb brown.

Serve with lemon wedges right away!

Notes:

1. Cook time: The fillets I used were about 2cm / 4/5" thick and they took about 6 minutes to cook.

2. Side suggestion - pictured in post with Creamy Mashed Cauliflower (low carb, super tasty alternative to mashed

potato!). This Garlic White Bean Mash In A Flash is also a handy quick side. For a quick meal, toast up some bread, grab a handful of leafy greens, drizzle with oil and lemon juice, pinch of salt and pepper - and voila!

44. SALTED SALMON

Prep Time: 8 hours

Cook Time: 8 minutes

Total Time: 8 hours 8 minutes

Ingredients

- 300g/10oz salmon fillets
- 15 g salt 5% of salmon weight
- 1 tbs sake

Instructions

Using a kitchen paper towel, pat the salmon fillets dry. Pour sake over salmon fillets and season with salt and pepper.
Season salmon fillets on both sides with salt.
Film the salmon fillets in a kitchen towel and cover with cling wrap.
Refrigerate the fillets for at least 7-8 hours or overnight.
Barbeque for 7-8 minutes in an oven set to 180 ° C.
Serve with simple steamed rice as a dipping sauce.

Notes

make bulk and store in freezer. It will be kept for a couple month in freezer. If you don't have cooking sake, it can be substituted by Chinese wine or dry cherry.

Nutrition

Calories: 223kcal | Protein: 29g | Fat: 9g | Saturated Fat: 1g | Cholesterol: 82mg | Sodium: 2973mg | Potassium: 735mg | Vitamin A: 60IU | Calcium: 18mg | Iron: 1.2mg

45. TROUT ALMONDINE

Total Time 25 minutes

Ingredients

- 2 (8-10 ounce) rainbow trout fillets
- salt and pepper
- 1/3 cup offlour
- 2 tbsp olive oil
- 2 tbsp salted butter
- 1/2 cups ofliced almonds
- juice from 1/2 lemon
- 2 tbsp chopped fresh parsley
- lemon wedges for serving

Instructions

Period the fish with salt and pepper before serving. On a rimmed plate or small bowl, spread flour out. Dredge both sides of the fish in flour and brush off any excess flour. In a big skillet, warm the oil over medium-high heat. Cook for 3 minutes with the fish skin side up. Make for another 2-3 minutes, or until the fillets are cooked through. Transfer the fish to a platter and cover with aluminum foil. Pour any remaining oil out of the skillet and wipe it clean with a paper towel. In a pan over medium heat, melt the butter. Make, stirring often, before the butter begins to brown and the almonds are aromatic, about 5-6 minutes. Remove the pan from the heat. mix the lemon juice and parsley in a mixing bowl.

On each serving plate, place 1 fish fillet. Half of the almond sauce should be spooned over each fillet. Serve with lemon slices on the side.

46. FISH NUGGETS

Ingredients

- 1 cup ofpanko (Japanese breadcrumbs)
- 1 tbspchopped fresh thym
- ½ tsp kosher salt
- ½ tsp freshly ground black pepper
- ½ cup ofall-purpose flou
- 2 tbsp water
- 1 large egg, lightly beaten
- 1 ½ pounds cod fillets, cut into 1-inch pieces
- Cooking spray
- ¼ cup ofcanola mayonnaise
- 1 tbspchopped dill pickle
- 2 tsp chopped fresh flat-leaf parsley
- ¼ tsp fresh lemon juice
- ¼ tsp Dijon mustard

Instructions

Preheat the oven to 400 degrees Fahrenheit.

In a big skillet,warm the oil over medium-high heat. Cook, stirring pan often, for 2 minutes or until golden brown, adding panko and thyme as needed. In a shallow dish, mix the panko mixture, salt, and pepper. In a separate shallow dish, add the flour. In a separate shallow dish, whisk together 2 tbsp water and the egg. Using the flour mixture, dredge the fish. Dredge in panko mixture after dipping in egg mixture. Arrange the fish on a baking sheet that has been sprayed with cooking spray in a single layer. Preheat oven to 400°F and bake fish for 12 minutes or until done.

In a mixing bowl, mix mayonnaise and additional ingredients; serve with nuggets.

Nutrition

Per Serving: 287 calories; fat 6.3g; saturated fat 0.6g; mono fat 2.9g; poly fat 2g; protein 31.3g; carbohydrates 22.5g; fiber 1.1g; cholesterol 126mg; iron 1.4mg; sodium 556mg; calcium 28mg.

47. CREAMY GARLIC BUTTER SALMON

PREP:5 MINS

COOK:20 MINS

TOTAL:25 MINS

INGREDIENTS

- 4 salmon fillets, skin off
- Salt and pepper, to season
- 2 tsp olive oil
- 2 tbsp butter
- 6 cloves garlic, finely diced
- 1 small yellow onion, diced
- 1/3 cup ofdry white wine
- 5 oz. sun dried tomato strips in oil in a container, drained
- 1 3/4 cups of half and half
- Salt and pepper, as need
- 3 cups of baby spinach leaves

- 1/2 cup offresh grated Parmesan cheese, (do not include for dairy free option)
- 1 tsp cornstarch (cornflour) mixed with 1 tbsp of water (optional)**
- 1 tbspfresh parsley chopped

INSTRUCTIONS

In a big skillet,warm the oil over medium-high heat.Period the salmon filets (or fish, if using) on both sides with salt and pepper, then sear in a hot skillet for 5 minutes on each side, flesh-side down first, or until cooked to your taste.Take the cooked chicken from the pan and set it aside.

Melt the butter in the pan juices that have remained. Fry the garlic until it is aromatic (about one minute). In a skillet, brown the onion in butter. Pour in the white wine and reduce by a small amount. Fry for 1-2 minutes to unleash the flavors of the sun dried tomatoes.

Reduce to a low heat setting, whisk in the half and half (or heavy cream), and cook to a slow simmer, stirring periodically. Season as need with salt and pepper.

Allow the spinach leaves to wilt in the sauce before mixing in the parmesan cheese. Allow the sauce to heat for another minute, or until the cheese has melted into the sauce. (To make a thicker sauce, pour the milk/cornstarch mixture into the center of the pan and continue to cook, stirring constantly, until the sauce thickens.)

Return the salmon to the pan with the parsley and the sauce spooned over each filet.

Serve with spaghetti, rice, or steamed vegetables as a dipping sauce.

NOTES

1/2 and 1/2 is an American product made from light cream and butter in equal parts. In place of half and half, you may use half light cream and half 2 percent milk. Use all heavy cream or all light cream as an alternative.

NUTRITION

Calories: 582kcal | Carbohydrates: 29g | Protein: 48g | Fat: 28g | Saturated Fat: 11g | Cholesterol: 136mg | Sodium: 476mg | Potassium: 2260mg | Fiber: 5g | Sugar: 18g | Vitamin A: 2960IU | Vitamin C: 27.5mg | Calcium: 235mg | Iron: 5.6mg

48. BAKED COD WITH TOMATOES AND ONIONS

Prep: 30 min

Inactive: 15 min

Cook: 20 min

Ingredients

- 1 (2 to 5-pound) line caught cod fillet with the skin-on
- 3 tbsp extra-virgin olive oil
- 1 tbsp+ 1 tsp kosher salt
- 11/2 tsp ground black pepper
- 5 large Roma plum tomatoes, stem ends removed, sliced lengthwise

- 1 1/2 cups of sliced yellow onions
- 2 tbsp minced garlic
- Olive Spread, recipe follows
- Cilantro sprigs, for garnish

Olive Spread:

- 1 tbsp minced shallots
- 2 cups of pitted brine-cured black olives
- 1 tbsp minced garlic
- 1 tbsp capers, drained
- 4 anchovy fillets
- 1 tbsp chopped parsley
- 2 tbsp lemon juice
- 1/4 cup of extra virgin olive oil
- 1/4 tsp freshly ground black pepper

Directions

Preheat oven to 400 degrees Fahrenheit.

In a big strainer, wash the fish under cold water. In a large non-reactive baking dish, cut 5 horizontal 3-inch slits on each side. 2 tbsp olive oil, 3 tsp kosher salt, and 1/2 tsp black pepper on both sides of the fish

Toss the sliced tomatoes, onions, garlic, 1 tbsp olive oil, 1 tsp kosher salt, and 1/2 tsp black pepper in a mixing bowl. Set away until you're ready.

In a roasting pan, place the fish skin side down. Apply a layer of olive spread to the top side of the fish. As scales, layer the tomatoes and cilantro flat on top of the tapenade, followed by the onions and garlic. Place the fish in the oven and bake for 20 minutes, or until the juices flow clear and the onions are crisping and slightly blackening along the edges.

Allow the fish to rest for 15 minutes after taking it from the oven. Serve the fish on a plate with cilantro sprigs as a garnish.

Spreading Olives:

1 1/2 cup ofyield

mix all of the ingredients in the bowl of a food processor and blend. Place in a mixing basin. Cover and leave away until required, or refrigerate in an airtight container for up to 3 days.

49. STEAMED MUSSELS WITH PEPPERS

Total Time

Prep: 30 min.

Cook: 10 min.

Ingredients

- 2 pound mussels, cleaned and with beards removed
- 1 jalapeno pepper, seeded and chopped
- 2 tbsp olive oil
- 3 garlic cloves, minced
- 1 bottle (8 ounces) clam juice
- 1/2 cup ofwhite wine or additional clam juice
- 1/3 cup ofchopped sweet red pepper
- 3 green onions, sliced

- 1/2 tsp dried oregano
- 1 bay leaf
- 2 tbsp minced fresh parsley
- 1/4 tsp salt
- 1/4 tsp pepper
- French bread baguette, sliced, optional

Directions

Any mussels that do not close should be discarded. Eliminate from the equation. Sauté jalapeño in oil in a large pan till tender. Cook for a additional minute after adding the garlic. mix the clam juice, wine, red pepper, green onions, oregano, and bay leaf in a mixing bowl.

Bring the water to a boil. Reduce the heat and add the mussels. Cook, covered, for 5-6 minutes, or until mussels open. Discard the bay leaf and any mussels that haven't opened. Add parsley, salt, and pepper as need. If preferred, serve with baguette pieces.

Note

When chopping hot peppers, use disposable gloves to avoid skin irritation from the oils. Keep your hands away from your face.

Nutrition

12 each: 293 calories, 12g fat, 65mg cholesterol, 931mg sodium, 12g carbohydrate , 28g protein.

50. CAJUN SALMON

Prep Time:5 mins

Cook Time:20 mins

Total Time:25 mins

Ingredients

- 1 lb. salmon fillet (skin on, boneless)
- 2 tbsp extra virgin olive oil
- 1/ tsp salt
- Seasoning Blend:
- 1 tsp Cajun or Creole seasoning
- 1 tsp garlic powder
- 1 tsp onion powder
- 1 tsp smoky paprika
- Black Pepper as need
- 1/4 lemon (zested, juiced)
- Italian parsley (for garnish)

Instructions

Preheat the oven to 425 degrees Fahrenheit. Seasonings should be mixd. Clean the fish by rinsing it and patting it dry. Place the salmon skin side down in the pan with 1 tbspof olive oil. Over the top of the salmon, drizzle the second tbspof olive oil.

Season with salt and massage spice into the surface of the fish.

Lemon juice and zest are sprinkled on top.

Preheat oven to 425°F and bake for 20-25 minutes.

Remove from the oven, sprinkle with parsley, and serve with more lemon zest and finely chopped parsley.

51. BAKED SALMON WITH GARLIC AND DIJON

Prep Time: 5 minutes

Cook Time: 15 minutes

Total Time: 20 minutes

Ingredients

- 1 1/2 pound filet de saumon
- 2 tbsp chopped fresh parsley
- 2 tbsp olive oil (mild, not extra virgin)
- 2 Tbsp fresh lemon juice
- 3 garlic cloves pressed
- 1/2 Tbsp Dijon mustard
- 1/2 tsp salt we use sea salt
- 1/8 tsp black pepper
- 1/2 Lemon sliced into 4 rings

Instructions

Warm the oven to 450 degrees Fahrenheit and prepare a rimmed baking sheet with parchment paper or foil. Cut the salmon into four halves and place them skin-side down on a parchment-lined baking sheet.

2 tbsp parsley, 2-3 crushed garlic cloves, 2 tbsp oil and 2 tbsp lemon juice, 1/2 tbsp Dijon, 1/2 tsp salt, and 1/8 tsp pepper in a small bowl

Spread the marinade to the top and sides of the salmon, then top with a slice of lemon on each piece.

Bake for 12-15 minutes at 450°F, or until just cooked through and flaky. Don't overcook the food.

Notes:

Place the salmon pieces on the wire basket, brush with the marinade, and air fry at 450°F for 6-7 minutes, or until cooked through.

Nutrition

Calories 314Calories from Fat 162% Daily Value*Fat 18g28%,Saturated Fat 3g19%,Cholesterol 94mg31%,Sodium 389mg17%,Potassium 872mg25%,Carbohydrates 3g1%

Fiber 1g4%,Sugar 1g1%,Protein 34g68%,Vitamin A 230IU5%

Vitamin C 13.3mg16%,Calcium 31mg3%,Iron 1.6mg9%

52. CHILI-GARLIC GLAZED SALMON

Prep:4 mins

Cook:7 mins

Total:11 mins

Ingredients

- 3 tbsp chili sauce with garlic (such as Hokan)
- 3 tbsp minced green onions (about 3 green onions)
- 1 ½ tbsp low-sugar orange marmalade
- ¾ tsp low-sodium soy sauce
- 4 (6-ounce) salmon fillets

Instructions

Preheat the oven to broil. In a small bowl, mix the first four ingredients; brush half of the chili sauce mixture over the fillets. Place the fillets on a baking sheet that has been sprayed with cooking spray, skin side down. 5 minutes under the broiler; brush with leftover chili sauce mixture. Broil for another 2 minutes, or until the salmon flakes readily when checked with a fork, or until desired doneness is reached.

Nutrition

Per Serving: 298 calories; calories from fat 40%; fat 13g; saturated fat 3.1g; mono fat 5.7g; poly fat 3.2g; protein 36.3g; carbohydrates 5.6g; fiber 0.5g; cholesterol 87mg; iron 0.6mg; sodium 171mg; calcium 23mg.

53. GARLIC BUTTER BAKED SALMON

PREP:10 MINS

COOK25: MINS

TOTAL:35 MINS

INGREDIENTS

- 1 pound (500 g) fingerling potatoes, halved
- 2 tbsp olive oil
- 1 1/2 tsp salt, divided
- 1/2 tsp cracked black pepper, divided
- 4 skinless salmon fillets
- 2 1/2 tbsp minced garlic, divided
- 2 tbsp fresh chopped parsley
- 1/3 cup offreshly squeezed lemon juice
- 1/2 cup ofmelted unsalted butter
- 3 bunches asparagus
- 2 tbsp dry white wine
- 1 lemon sliced to garnish

INSTRUCTIONS

Warm the oven to 400 degrees Fahrenheit. Stir the potatoes with the oil before serving, 1/2 tbspof garlic, 1/2 tsp salt, and 1/4 tsp pepper on a large rimmed baking sheet. Spread them in an equal layer and roast for 15 minutes, or until they soften and brown slightly.

Place the potatoes on one side and the salmon in the center of the sheet pan. 1 1/2 tbsp minced garlic and 2 tbsp parsley should be equally applied to the fish. On the opposite side of the pan, add the asparagus.

1/4 cup of lemon juice and 1/4 cup of melted butter are mixed together and poured over the fish and asparagus. With the remaining salt and pepper, season everything.

Return to the oven and bake until the potatoes are golden and fork-tender and the salmon is opaque all the way through, about 20 minutes (about 10 minutes). Broil for burnt edges in the last 2 minutes if desired.

Meanwhile, mix the remaining butter, garlic, and lemon juice with the wine in a small bowl (or chicken stock). Serve with lemon slices, vegetables, and fish!

NUTRITION

513 calories | 19 grams of carbohydrates | 37 grams of protein | 38 grams of fat | 15 grams of saturated fat | 154 milligrams of cholesterol | 970 milligrams of sodium | 1549 milligrams of potassium | 5 grams of fiber | 2 grams of sugar

54. SIMPLE GARLIC SHRIMP

Prep:15 mins

Cook:10 mins

Total:25 mins

Ingredient

- 1 ½ tbsp olive oil
- 1 pound shrimp, peeled and deveined
- salt as need
- 6 cloves garlic, finely minced
- ¼ tsp red pepper flakes
- 3 tbsp lemon juice
- 1 tbspcaper brine
- 1 ½ tsp cold butter
- ⅓ cup ofchopped Italian flat leaf parsley, divided
- 1 ½ tbsp cold butter
- water, as needed

Instructions

In a big skillet,warm the vegetable oil over high heat until it just begins to smoke. Cook for 1 minute without stirring after placing shrimp in an equal layer on the bottom of the pan. Season shrimp with salt and cook, stirring constantly, until they become pink, approximately 1 minute.

Make and stir for 1 minute after adding the garlic and red pepper flakes. mix the lemon juice, caper brine, 1 1/2 tsp chilled butter, and half of the parsley in a mixing bowl.Make for 1 minute, or before butter has melted, then reduce heat to low and whisk in 1 1/2 tsp cold butter.Make and stir for 2 to 3 minutes, or until all of the butter has melted and the shrimp are pink and opaque.

Remove the shrimp with a slotted spoon and place them in a bowl; continue to boil the butter sauce for another 2 minutes, adding water 1 tsp at a time if it becomes too thick. As need, season with salt.

Serve the shrimp with the pan sauce on top. Serve with the remaining flat-leaf parsley as a garnish.

Nutrition

Per Serving: 196 calories; protein 19.1g; carbohydrates 2.9g; fat 12g; cholesterol 188.1mg; sodium 243.7mg.

55. SPICY OVEN FRIED CATFISH

Prep Time: 15 minutes

Cook Time: 25 minutes

Total Time: 40 minutes

Ingredients

- Non-stick olive oil spray
- 2/3 cup ofyellow cornmeal
- 1/4 cup ofall-purpose flour
- 1 1/2-2 tsp seasoned salt
- 1/2 tsp black pepper
- 1/2 tsp cayenne pepper
- 1/2 tsp lemon pepper
- 1/4 tsp paprika
- 2 large eggs
- 2 tsp hot sauce
- 1 pound catfish fillets cut into smaller pieces

Instructions

Preheat the oven to 425°F. Line a roasting sheet with parchment paper that has been thoroughly coated with non-stick olive oil spray.

mix cornmeal, flour, salt, pepper, cayenne, lemon pepper, and paprika in a brown bag or ziploc bag and shake well.

Whisk together eggs and spicy sauce in a deep pie plate or big shallow basin.

Toss each fish in the cornmeal breading to coat, then dab both sides in beaten eggs, then return to the cornmeal breading and shake freely to coat. Place the fillet on the baking sheet that has been coated. Carry on with the rest of the fillets in the same manner.

Using non-stick baking spray, liberally coat the tops of each fillet, making sure the fish is thoroughly covered. Depending on the thickness of the fillets, bake for 25-30 minutes, or until golden brown on the outside but still juicy on the interior.

Take the fish from of the pan and set away for 5 minutes to cool before serving with lemon and parsley.

56. HALIBUT WITH BALSAMIC GLAZE

Prep: 10 min

Inactive: 30 min

Cook: 15 min

Ingredient

- 1/2 cup ofbalsamic vinegar
- 2-3 tablespoons honey (based on how sweet you want it)
- 3 tbsp vegetable oil
- 2 garlic cloves, minced
- 4 (6-ounce) halibut fillets
- Nonstick cooking spray

Directions

In a mixing bowl, mix the vinegar, honey, oil, and garlic. In an 8-inch square baking dish, arrange the halibuts. Pour the marinade over the fish, making sure it is fully covered. After covering, chill for at least 30 minutes and up to 4 hours.

Preheat the oven to broil. Using foil, line the bottom and sides of a baking sheet. Using nonstick frying spray, coat the foil. Remove the fillets from the marinade and place them on the baking sheet, reserving the marinade. Fill a heavy small saucepan halfway with the marinade. Broil the fillets for 12 minutes, or until they are just cooked through and caramelized on top.

Meanwhile, bring the marinade to a boil and cook, stirring constantly, until it thickens slightly and becomes syrupy, about 15 minutes. If desired, drain any extra oil from the sauce.

Place the fillets on serving plates.Present with the sauce slurped over and across the fillets.

57. LEMON PEPPER SALMON

PREP:10 mins

COOK:15 mins

TOTAL:30 mins

Ingredients

- 2 pound side of salmon boneless wild caught if possible
- 10 sprigs of fresh thyme optional, but delicious
- 2 medium lemons + additional for serving
- 2 tbsp extra virgin olive oil
- 1 tsp kosher salt
- 1/2 tsp newly crushed black pepper + more if needed
- finely chopped fresh herbs of choice

Instructions

Take the salmon from the refrigerator and set it aside for 10 minutes to come to room temperature while you prepare the rest of the ingredients. Preheat the oven to 375 degrees Fahrenheit. Using a big piece of aluminum foil, line a rimmed baking sheet large enough to contain your piece of salmon.If you don't want the salmon to touch the foil, use a sheet of parchment paper on top of it.

Add a little coating of baking spray to the foil, then place 5 thyme sprigs down the center. Half of one of the lemons should be cut into thin slices and placed down the center. On top of it, place the salmon.

Drizzle the olive oil over the fish. Over the fish, zest the second lemon and season with salt and pepper. On top of the salmon, scatter the remaining thyme and lemon segments. Pour the juice from the zested lemon over the top.

Fold the aluminum foil sides up and over the top of the salmon to completely cover it. Place a second sheet of foil on top and fold the edges under to make a sealed packet if your first piece isn't big enough. Allow a small amount of space within the foil for air to flow.

Bake for 15-20 minutes, or until the thickest portion of the salmon is almost entirely cooked through. Depending on the thickness of your fish, the cooking time will vary. Check several minutes early if your side is thinner (about 1-inch thick) to ensure your salmon does not overcook. It may take much longer if your item is really thick (12 inches or more).

Remove the salmon from the oven and carefully unwrap the foil to expose the whole top of the fish (be careful of hot steam). Change the oven setting to broil, then return the salmon to the oven and broil for 3 minutes, or until the top is slightly brown and the fish is thoroughly cooked through. To avoid overcooking the salmon, keep an eye on it as it broils. Take the salmon out of the oven. If it still seems underdone, wrap the foil around it again and let it aside for a few minutes. Allow it to sit for a short time—salmon may rapidly go from "not done" to "over done." It's ready when it readily flakes with a fork.

Cut the fish into pieces to serve. As desired, top with more fresh herbs or a squeeze of lemon.

Notes

Because reheated salmon might dry up, this recipe is best eaten the day it is prepared.
STORAGE: Refrigerate baked lemon pepper salmon for 1 to 2 days in an airtight storage container.
TO REHEAT: I recommend reheating individual pieces in a pan or in the microwave on low power. Before reheating the salmon, let it to come to room temperature.

REMOVE IT FROM THE SKIN AND FREEZE IT FOR UP TO TWO MONTHS IN AN AIRTIGHT CONTAINER. Allow it to defrost overnight in the refrigerator.

Nutrition

SERVING: 1(of 6), about 6 ounces each,CALORIES: 268kcal,CARBOHYDRATES: 4g,PROTEIN: 31g,FAT: 14g,SATURATED FAT: 2g,CHOLESTEROL: 83mg,POTASSIUM: 801mg,FIBER: 1g,SUGAR: 1g,VITAMIN A: 140IU,VITAMIN C: 22mg,CALCIUM: 34mg,IRON: 2mg

58. CRISPY TILAPIA

READY IN: 16mins

INGREDIENTS

- 3lbs tilapia fillets, about 10
- 1/3cup offlour, for dusting fish
- 1egg
- 1/2cup ofbuttermilk
- 1/2cup offlour
- 1/2cup ofyellow cornmeal
- saltpepper
- 1/tsp baking soda
- 1/2tsp baking powder
- 2tbsp Old Bay Seasoning
- canola oil, to cover bottom of big pan

Directions

Season the fish with salt and pepper. 1/3 cup offlour, dusted on fillets

In a single bow, mix the egg and buttermilk.

In a separate basin, mix flour, corn meal, baking soda, baking powder, and Old Bay.

All of the floured fish should be dipped in the egg and then into the flour mixture.

In a big pan,warm the oil to medium-high.

Roast for 2 minutes on each side before flipping.

As soon as you take the pan from the heat, season it with salt.

Three batches should be completed.

59. CRISP FRIED PRAWNS

Prep Time: 10 mins

Cook Time: 20 mins

Total Cook Time: 30 mins

INGREDIENTS

- 12 prawns (bombed)
- 2 Tbsp wine
- 2 tablespoons soy sauce
- 1 teaspoon of sugar
- 2 tsp onion sauce
- 1 tsp ginger sauce
- 2 eggs, whisked
- 2 tbsp corn starch
- For roasting sauce, 25 gram flour oil
- 1 tablespoon of oil
- 1/2 t
- easpoon garlic, chopped
- 1 tsp red chilies, diced
- 2 tbsp spring onion, chopped

- 2 tablespoons corn flour
- 1 teaspoon of sugar
- 150 milliliters of water
- Tomato ketchup, 3 tbsp
- 1 tablespoon soy sauce
- 1 tablespoon of Worcestershire sauce
- 1 tablespoon sesame oil

Directions

mix prawns, soy sauce, wine, sugar, garlic, ginger, and eggs in a mixing bowl. Allow it to marinate for 30 minutes. mix corn flour and flour in a mixing bowl. Toss to coat. Then deep fry till crisp and golden brown in hot oil. Serve it with a dipping sauce. To make the sauce:

Stir-fry the chilies, garlic, and spring onions in a wok for 30 seconds.

Except for the sesame oil, mix the remaining ingredients.

Before adding sesame oil, stir to thicken. Serve with prawns on the side.

60. PRAWNS WITH GARLIC BUTTER

Preparation time: 30 mins

Cooking time: 10 mins

Ingredients

- 1 tbsp olive oil
- 50g/2oz butter
- 12 large raw prawns
- 2 garlic cloves, crushed
- salt and freshly ground black pepper
- small handful parsley, chopped

DIRECTIONS

Warm the oil and butter in a wok or a big pan. Stir in the prawns and garlic until thoroughly mixd. Stir-fry for 4–5 minutes, or until the prawns are pink and cooked through.

Season as need with salt and freshly ground black pepper, then top with chopped parsley. Serve right away.

61. GRILLED GARLIC SHRIMP WITH SAFFRON

READY IN: 2hrs 10mins

INGREDIENTS

- 1/3cup ofextra virgin olive oil
- 2pinches saffron threads
- 2tbsp fresh lime juice
- 2garlic cloves, finely minced
- 20raw jumbo shrimp

DIRECTIONS

Whisk together the vegetable oil, saffron, lime juice, and garlic in a medium nonreactive bowl. Toss in the shrimp to coat.

Refrigerate for 2 hours after covering.

Preheat the grill to medium-high.

Allow the excess marinade to drip off before threading the shrimp onto four metal skewers.

Grill until the center is barely opaque, about 2 minutes per side.

62. HEALTHY LEMON VEGETABLE & FISH FOIL PACKETS

Prep Time:10 mins

Cook Time:15 mins

Total Time:25 mins

Ingredients

- 1 medium onion sliced
- 1/2 pound green beans trimmed
- 1 tbspolive oil
- salt & pepper as need
- 4 fish fillets tilapia, salmon, cod, etc.
- 2 tbsp butter melted
- 3 cloves garlic minced
- 1/2 tsp each salt and pepper
- 1/4 tsp red pepper flakes optional
- 1 lemon thinly sliced into 8 pieces

Instructions

Cut four 15-inch-long strips of heavy-duty aluminum foil (if using regular aluminum foil, double it).

Divide the onions and green beans among the foil pieces, starting with the onions and ending with the green beans.

Season the veggies with salt and pepper after drizzling them with olive oil.

On top of each veggie mound, place a fish fillet. mix the butter, garlic, salt, pepper, and optional red pepper flakes in a mixing bowl and spread equally over the fish.

Wrap foil over each pile of fish and veggies, folding edges to seal firmly, then top with two thin slices of lemon.

Preheat the grill to medium-high heat and lay the packets immediately on the grill. Cook 1/2-inch fillets for 15 minutes, covered (until fish flakes easily with a fork). Cook thicker fillets for a little longer if necessary.

To bake, place packets on a baking sheet and bake for about 20 minutes, or until done, at 400 degrees.

Carefully unwrap packets, being mindful of steam, and serve on separate plates in the envelopes.

Notes

Asparagus, thinly sliced carrots, sliced sweet peppers, chopped cabbage, or kale (or whatever else you want!) can be used in place of green beans.

Nutrition

Serving: 1packet | Calories: 228kcal | Carbohydrates: 8.9g | Protein: 23.7g | Fat: 11.9g | Saturated Fat: 5.2g | Cholesterol: 65mg | Sodium: 667mg | Fiber: 3.1g | Sugar: 2.4g

63. ASIAN SALMON FOIL-PACK DINNER

Prep:5 mins

Cook:30 mins

Total:35 mins

Ingredients

- 1 (6 ounce) salmon fillet
- 2 tbsp honey
- 1 clove garlic, minced
- 1 tsp soy sauce
- 1 tsp rice vinegar
- 1 tsp sriracha sauce
- ½ tsp sesame oil
- ½ tsp refrigerated ginger paste
- 1 cups ofugar snap peas
- ¼ cups ofliced mushrooms
- 1 tbspsweet chili sauce

Instructions

Warm oven to 400 degrees Fahrenheit (200 degrees C). On a level work surface, place a piece of aluminum foil. Place the salmon filet in the foil's center. In a small bowl, mix the honey, garlic, soy sauce, rice vinegar, sriracha sauce, sesame oil, and ginger paste. Pour the sauce over the fish.

In a separate bowl, mix the snap peas, mushrooms, and sweet chili sauce. Arrange the vegetables in a circle around the fish. To make a sealed packet, fold the foil over on itself.

Bake for 25 minutes in a preheated oven until salmon flakes easily with a fork. Carefully open the packet to reveal the salmon, then broil on low for 5 minutes, or until the glaze has caramelized.

Nutrition

Per Serving: 555 calories; protein 34.9g; carbohydrates 60.9g; fat 18.9g; cholesterol 82.5mg; sodium 779.7mg. Full Nutrition

64. CHICKEN BROCCOLI STIR FRY

Prep Time: 15 minutes

Cook Time: 15 minutes

Total Time: 30 minutes

Ingredients

- 1 lb chicken breast, cut into 3/4" pieces
- 2 Tbsp cooking oil, divided
- 1 lb broccoli cut into florets
- 1 little yellow onion sliced into strips
- 1/2 lb white button mushrooms sliced

Stir Fry Sauce Ingredients:

- 2/3 cup oflow sodium chicken broth
- 3 Tbsp low sodium soy sauce, or added as need
- 2 Tbsp light brown sugar packed
- 1 Tbsp corn starch
- 1 Tbsp sesame oil
- 1 tsp fresh ginger peeled and grated
- 1 tsp garlic grated
- 1/4 tsp black pepper + more to season chicken

Instructions

Whisk together all of the sauce ingredients in a small bowl to dissolve the sugar and corn starch (warm broth will help dissolve the sugar faster). Set aside the sauce. Season generously with pepper and cut chicken into small bite-sized pieces (no more than 3/4" thick). Over medium-high heat, heat a big heavy skillet or wok. 1 tbsp. olive oil Add the chicken in a single layer to the pan and leave it alone for 1 minute to achieve a nice sear, then stir fry for another 5 minutes or until golden brown and cooked through, then transfer to a bowl and cover loosely to keep warm.

1 tbspoil, broccoli florets, sliced onion, and sliced mushrooms in the same skillet. Reduce warm to medium/low after 3 minutes, or until mushrooms are softened and broccoli is crisp-tender.

Give the sauce a brief toss to cut ties any clumps of starch, then pour it all over the veggies. Simmer for 3-4 minutes, or before the sauce has thickened and the flavors of the garlic and ginger have mellowed. Add a spoonful of water at a time to thin the sauce. Return the chicken to the pan and toss for another 30 seconds, or until well warm. If needed, season with additional soy sauce and serve over hot rice.

Nutrition

Calories 325Calories from Fat 126% Daily Value*,Fat 14g22%,Saturated Fat 2g13%,Cholesterol 73mg24%,Sodium 586mg25%,Potassium 1039mg30%,Carbohydrates 21g7%

Fiber 4g17%,Sugar 10g11%,Protein 31g62%,Vitamin A 740IU15%,Vitamin C 105mg127%,Calcium 68mg7%,Iron 2mg11%.

65. CHICKEN FAJITAS

Prep Time:10 minutes

Cook Time:20 minutes

Marinating Time:1 hour

INGREDIENTS

- 1 1/2 lbs sliced boneless and skinless chicken breasts
- 1/4 cup ofolive oil
- 1/3 cup oflime juice
- 1 tsp sugar
- 1 1/4 tsp salt
- 1/4 tsp ground cumin
- 2 cloves garlic minced
- 1/4 cup ofwater
- 1 1/2 tsp smoked paprika
- 1 tsp onion powder
- 1 1/2 tbsp chili powder

For the fajitas

- 2 tsp olive oil
- 1 thinly sliced yellow onion
- 3 thinly sliced
- bell peppers (red, orange, yellow, or a mix of colors)
- salt as need
- 2 tbsp chopped cilantro
- tortillas, guacamole, sour cream, cheese, salsa etc for serving

INSTRUCTIONS

Combine 1/4 cup olive oil, lime juice, sugar, salt, cumin, garlic, water, smoked paprika, onion powder, and chili powder
in a gallon-sized resealable bag or large mixing bowl.joint all of the ingredients in a large mixing bowl and whisk until fully smooth.
Combine the chicken, onions, and peppers in a large mixing basin. Allow at least 1 hour, but up to 8 hours, for cooling.

To make the fajitas

, combine all of the ingredients in a large mixing bowl.
2 tbsp olive oil, heated in a large pan over medium heat
In a mixing bowl, combine the chicken and peppers. Cook for 6-8 minutes, stirring periodically, or until chicken is cooked through and vegetables are soft. Season with salt as need
ed if desired.
After sprinkling cilantro over the fajitas, serve with tortillas and toppings of your choice.

NOTES

Preheat a grill or an indoor grill pan to medium heat for grilled fajitas. If you're using an outside barbecue, use a grilling basket.

Cook, stirring periodically, for 6-8 minutes with the chicken and veggies.

Place the chicken, peppers, and onions on a sheet pan that has been sprayed with cooking spray. Broil for 8-10 minutes, stirring every now and again.

NUTRITION

Calories: 226kcal | Carbohydrates: 8g | Protein: 20g | Fat: 13g | Saturated Fat: 3g | Cholesterol: 68mg | Sodium: 582mg | Potassium: 605mg | Fiber: 2g | Sugar: 4g | Vitamin A: 2700IU | Vitamin C: 81.7mg | Calcium: 43mg | Iron: 2.6mg

66. CHICKEN HASH

Prep:30 mins

Cook:1 hr

Total:1 hr 30 mins

Ingredients

- 3 tbsp vegetable oil
- 1 pound bone-in chicken thighs
- Salt and pepper
- ½ cup of low-sodium chicken broth
- 1 ½ pounds potatoes, peeled, cut into 1/2-inch dice
- ½ medium red onion, diced
- ½ medium green bell pepper, seeded and diced

- 2 scallions, chopped, divided into white and green sections
- 1 clove garlic, minced
- ½ tsp dried thyme
- ½ tsp paprika

Directions

In a pan over medium-high heat, warm 1 tbsp of oil. Period the chicken with salt and pepper before serving. Cook for 10 minutes, rotating once. Away any remaining fat. Pour in the broth, cover, and simmer for 35 minutes on low heat. Take the chicken and set it aside to cool. Meat should be shredded. Take the fat from the cooking liquid and set aside. Fill a saucepan halfway with salted water and bring to a boil. Drain after 5 minutes of cooking. In a skillet over medium-high heat, warm the remaining oil. For 5 minutes, sauté potatoes, onion, bell pepper, and white portions of scallions. Sauté for 4 minutes with garlic, thyme, paprika, 1 tsp salt, and 1/2 tsp pepper. Add the chicken and make for 3 minutes, adding additional liquid as required. Before serving, top with scallion greens.

Nutrition

Per Serving: 441 calories; fat 23g; saturated fat 5g; protein 24g; carbohydrates 34g; fiber 3g; cholesterol 95mg; sodium 397mg.

67. CHICKEN NUGGETS

Total: 25 min

Prep: 15 min

Cook: 10 min

Ingredients

- 1/2 cup ofall-purpose flour
- 1 tsp granulated garlic
- Kosher salt and ground black pepper
- 2 chicken breasts, armless and chicken skinless, cut into 1 1/2-inch pieces
- 1 cup ofprepared breadcrumbs
- 1 large egg
- 1 cup ofvegetable oil

Directions

Season the flour with the garlic, 1 tsp salt, and 1/4 tsp pepper in a resealable plastic bag. Toss the chicken pieces with the flour in the bag to coat them (work in batches).Period the breadcrumbs with salt and pepper and set aside on a rimmed plate.

In a medium blending bowl, whisk together the egg and 1 tbspwater. Take a piece of chicken from the flour, dip it into the egg mixture, then into the breadcrumbs, gently pressing the crumbs into the chicken, and place it on a plate. Rep with the remaining chicken pieces.

In a big frying pan, heat the vegetable oil over medium-high heat. Brown the chicken pieces in the pan for about 8 minutes total. Transfer the chicken nuggets to a paper towel-lined plate using a spatula. Season with salt and pepper while still hot, then serve.

68. CHICKEN THIGHS

Prep: 5 mins

Cook: 35 mins

Total: 40 mins

INGREDIENTS

- 2 lb chicken thighs bone-in skin-on
- 1 tsp salt or as need
- 1 tsp black pepper or as need
- Sauce
- 2 tbsp olive oil
- 1 tbsp whole grain dijon mustard
- 1 tbsp mustard
- 2 tbsp honey
- 6 cloves garlic minced
- ¼ tsp red pepper flakes

INSTRUCTIONS

Preheat the oven to 425 degrees Fahrenheit.
Period the chicken thighs generously with salt and pepper in a mixing basin.

In a small mixing bowl, mix all of the sauce ingredients. Toss the thighs in the sauce till fully coated.

Transfer the chicken thighs, along with any leftover sauce, to a 9_13 inch baking dish. There's no need to grease the pan.Warm the oven to 350°F and bake the chicken thighs for 35 minutes, or until the internal temperature reaches 165°F and the skin is crispy.

Before serving, transfer the chicken to a serving platter, cover with aluminum foil, and let aside for 10 minutes.

NOTES

You may also use boneless, skinless chicken thighs, but they will roast quickly, taking only 20 to 25 minutes in the oven.

To choose whether or not use the honey mustard glaze is totally up to you. Simply season the thighs with salt and pepper, sprinkle a couple tbsp of olive oil in the baking dish, and bake as directed for a simpler chicken thigh recipe.

This oven cooked chicken can keep in the fridge for up to 3 days if properly kept or wrapped. To lengthen the shelf life, I recommend freezing it. The chicken will keep in the freezer for 4-6 months if packed in an airtight container.

Nutrition

Serving: 1thighCalories: 403kcal (20%)Carbohydrates: 8g (3%)Protein: 25g (50%)Fat: 30g (46%)Saturated Fat: 7g (44%)Cholesterol: 148mg (49%)Sodium: 563mg (24%)Potassium: 322mg (9%)Fiber: 1g (4%)Sugar: 6g (7%)Vitamin A: 143IU (3%)Vitamin C: 1mg (1%)Calcium: 18mg (2%)Iron: 1mg (6%)

69. CHICKEN PARMESAN

Prep:25 mins

Cook:20 mins

Additional:15 mins

Total:1 hr

Ingredients

- 4 skinless, boneless chicken breast halves
- salt and freshly ground black pepper as need
- 2 eggs
- 1 cup ofpanko bread crumbs, or more as needed
- ½ cup ofgrated Parmesan cheese
- 2 tbsp all-purpose flour, or more if needed
- 1 cup ofolive oil for frying
- ½ cup ofprepared tomato sauce
- ¼ cup offresh mozzarella, cut into small cubes
- ¼ cup ofchopped fresh basil
- ½ cup ofgrated provolone cheese
- ¼ cup ofgrated Parmesan cheese
- 1 tbspolive oil

Instructions

Warm the oven to 450 degrees Fahrenheit (230 degrees C). Place chicken breasts on a sturdy, flat surface between two sheets of thick plastic (resealable freezer bags work nicely). Using the smooth side of a meat mallet, pound the chicken to a thickness of

1/2 inch. Season the chicken with salt and pepper as need.In a shallow bowl, whisk all together eggs and set aside.

In a separate bowl, mix bread crumbs and 1/2 cup ofParmesan cheese; set aside.

In a sifter or sieve, sift the flour and evenly cover both sides of the chicken breasts.

Using beaten eggs, coat the flour-coated chicken breasts. Place the breast in the breadcrumb mixture and press the crumbs into both sides of the breast. Rep with the other breast. Breaded chicken breasts should be set aside for about 15 minutes.

In a large pan, heat 1 cup ofolive oil over medium-high heat until it shimmers.Make the chicken until golden brown on both sides, about 2 minutes each side. In the oven, the chicken will finish cooking.

Place the chicken in a baking dish and pour about 1/3 cup oftomato sauce over each breast. Equal quantities of mozzarella cheese, fresh basil, and provolone cheese are layered on each chicken breast. Drizzle 1 tbspolive oil over the top and sprinkle 1 to 2 tbsp Parmesan cheese on top. 15 to 20 minutes in a preheated oven, bake until cheese is browned and bubbling and chicken breasts are no longer pink in the center. At least 165 degrees F should be read on an instant-read thermometer placed into the middle (74 degrees C).

Note:

For a better outcome, use high-quality prepared tomato sauce. You may replace the basil with pesto or dried Italian herbs of your choosing, or leave it out completely. If you're using fresh mozzarella, instead of shredding it, cut it into cubes.

Nutrition

Per Serving: 471 calories; protein 42.1g; carbohydrates 24.8g; fat 24.9g; cholesterol 186.7mg; sodium 840.3mg. Full Nutrition.

70. PAN-ROASTED CHICKEN AND VEGETABLES

Prep: 15 min

Bake: 45 min.

Ingredients

- 2 pounds red potatoes (about 6 medium), cut into 3/4-inch pieces
- 1 large onion, coarsely chopped
- 2 tbsp olive oil
- 3 garlic cloves, minced
- 1-1/4 tsp salt, divided
- 1 tsp dried rosemary, crushed, divided
- 3/4 tsp pepper, divided
- 1/2 tsp paprika
- 6 bone-in chicken thighs (about 2-1/4 pounds), skin removed
- 6 cups of fresh baby spinach (about 6 ounces)

Directions

Preheat the oven to 425 degrees Fahrenheit. Toss potatoes, onion, oil, garlic, 3/4 tsp salt, 1/2 tsp rosemary, and 1/2 tsp pepper in a large mixing basin to coat. Place in a 15x10x1-inch baking pan that has been sprayed with cooking spray.

mix paprika, the remaining salt, rosemary, and pepper in a small bowl. Toss the chicken with the paprika mixture and place it on top of the veggies. Roast for 35-40 minutes, or until a thermometer placed in the chicken registers 170°-175° and the veggies are just tender.

Transfer the chicken to a serving plate and set aside to keep warm. Add spinach to the veggies as a garnish. Roast for another 8-10 minutes, or before the veggies are soft and the spinach has wilted. Toss the veggies together and serve with the chicken.

71. CHICKEN WINGS

Prep: 5 minutes

Cook: 45 minutes

Total: 50 minutes

Ingredients

- 1/3 cup offlour
- 2 tbsp paprika
- 1 tsp garlic powder
- 1 tsp black pepper
- 1 tsp salt
- 3 tbsp butter
- 10 chicken wingettes just means tips removed, thawed

Instructions

Preheat the oven to 425 degrees Fahrenheit. Using foil, line a baking pan. Spread the butter over the foil; there's no need to melt it ahead of time, but you may if you like.

 mix flour, paprika, garlic powder, salt, and pepper in a medium mixing basin.

Place each wing on the baking sheet, completely coated in the flour mixture on both sides. Ensure that the butter bits are equally distributed throughout the wings.

Preheat oven to 350°F and bake wings for 30 minutes.

Turn the wings over and bake for another 15 minutes, or until crispy and cooked through.

Garnish with your favorite dipping sauce with fresh parsley, if desired.

Enjoy!

72. CRUMBED CHICKEN TENDERLOINS

Prep:15 mins

Cook:12 mins

Total:27 mins

Ingredients

- 1 egg
- ½ cup ofdry bread crumbs
- 2 tbsp vegetable oil
- 8 chicken tenderloins

Instructions

Warm your air fryer to 350°F (175 degrees C). In a small bowl, whisk the egg. In a second bowl, mix bread crumbs and oil until the mixture is loose and crumbly.

Shake off any excess egg after dipping each chicken tenderloin in the egg. Make sure the chicken is evenly and completely coated in the crumb mixture.In the steamer basket, add the chicken loin chops.Make for 12 minutes, or until the center is no longer pink. At least 165 degrees F should be read on an instant-read thermometer placed into the middle (74 degrees C).

Note:

If preferred, butter can be used instead of the vegetable oil.

Nutrition

Per Serving: 253 calories; protein 26.2g; carbohydrates 9.8g; fat 11.4g; cholesterol 109mg; sodium 170.7mg. Full Nutrition

73. GENERAL TSO'S CHICKEN

Prep: 15 mins

Cook: 10 mins

Ingredients

- 3 tbsp mild or even all soy sauce
- 1 tablespoon of hoisin sauce
- 1 tbsp acid (rice)
- 2 tsp chilli paste , any
- 1 tsp sesame oil toasted preferably
- 3 tbsp brown sugar
- 1 tbsp cornflour/cornstarch
- 3/4 cup ofchicken stock/broth , low sodium

CHICKEN:

- 600g/ 1.4 lb chicken thighs , boneless skinless, cut into 2.5cm / 1" pieces (breast / tenderloin - Note 2)
- 1 tsp ginger , finely grated
- 1 tsp garlic ,finely grated
- 1 cup ofcornflour/cornstarch (Note 5)
- 1 - 4 cups of oil, for frying (peanut, vegetable or canola; Note 4)

STIR FRY SAUCE:

- 2 tbsp oil (peanut, vegetable or canola)
- 2 tsp ginger , finely chopped (Note 3)
- 2 cloves garlic , finely chopped (Note 3)

- 1/2 tsp red chilli flakes (red pepper flakes)

GARNISHES (AT LEAST 1 RECOMMENDED):

- Finely sliced green onion
- Sesame seeds

Instructions

To make the sauce-marinade, mix the soy sauce, hoisin sauce, vinegar, chili, and sesame oil.

Take 2 tbsp of the Sauce-Marinade and mix with the chicken. Mix in the ginger and garlic with the chicken, then marinate for 30 minutes.

Toss the cornflour into the chicken and toss to coat, making sure that the pieces are separated so that they are evenly covered.

Remove extra cornflour by sifting it into a strainer and shaking it out (or grab handfuls, shake so cornflour falls through your fingers).

Finish the sauce by adding sugar and cornflour to the leftover Sauce-Marinade (from Step 1) After that, add the chicken stock and mix again.

Heat 2 cm/4/5" oil to 200°C/390°F in a deep skillet (or large pot - whatever you're comfortable with). See Note 4 for more information on how to use less.

Cook for 3 minutes, rotating halfway through, or until golden and crispy. Drain on a platter lined with paper towels.

Clean / new skillet: Take the skillet from the heat and discard the oil. Alternatively, use a second big skillet.

Stir Fry Sauce: In a large pan over medium heat, heat the oil. Sauté garlic, ginger, and chili flakes for 30 seconds, or until light golden. Add the sauce, bring to a low simmer, and stir occasionally until it thickens enough to form a trail over the bottom of the pan.

Toss! Toss in the chicken and toss quickly to coat - the faster you are, the crispier the chicken will be! Transfer to a serving platter, decorate, and serve with your favorite rice.

Notes:

1. All-purpose or light soy sauce is necessary here. It's acceptable to use either, but don't use dark soy sauce (labeled as such) because it will overpower the flavor and turn the sauce too dark. You may learn something about various soy sauces here.
2. Chicken thigh is the finest choice since it will stay juicy on the inside. Breast is prone to overcooking and drying out, and deep frying is especially dangerous because most people aren't familiar with deep or semi-deep frying.
BREAST & TENDELLIN - If you absolutely want to use breast, tenderize it a little to give yourself some leeway to overcook it without drying it out. mix 1/4 tsp baking soda (bi-carb) with the marinade sauce and leave to marinate for 1 hour or overnight. This is a simplified version of the Chinese Restaurant Method of Tenderizing Chicken (using less bicarb and marinating for longer so you don't have to rinse it).

3. For the chicken marinade, use a microplane or equivalent fine grater to grate the garlic and ginger. Using a knife, finely chop the ingredients for stir frying. When using a garlic press or microplane grater, the garlic and ginger become excessively wet and paste-like, and when stir-fried, they burn quickly.

4. Amount of oil to use - it's ideal to use enough oil to cover the chicken halfway up the side (from the pan's bottom) so you only have to turn it once to achieve excellent crispy chicken (ie. shallow frying). You may also add extra oil, to the point that the chicken is bobbing in it, for a more uniform crispy coating all over (ie. deep frying).

If you don't want to fry and want to use as little oil as possible, simply coat the bottom of the pan with oil and cook over medium-high heat. Cook the chicken for a total of 3 - 4 minutes, rotating to crisp up as many sides as possible (this is laborious, which is why I shallow fry!)

5. Cornflour for coating - I know 1 cup of cornflour for 600g/1.2 pound of chicken seems excessive. To ensure that there is enough to adequately coat the chicken all over using the mixing then shaking off procedure, I err on the liberal side. Due to the cornflour clumping from the chicken fluids / marinade, you lose quite a bit. If you toss thoroughly and fast, you might probably get away with 3/4 cup. You could also use 1/2 cup of if you dipped each piece of chicken in cornflour one at a time and brushed off the excess.

6. Sesame oil - toasted sesame oil is darker in color and has a stronger flavor than untoasted sesame oil (which is yellow). Toasted sesame oil is the most common kind available in Australia; untoasted sesame oil is more difficult to come by.

7. Refrigeration and reheating - Keeps for up to 5 days in the fridge. The chicken will not be crispy if reheated (add a little water if sauce is too thick). Even so, everyone who reheated their leftovers raved about it!

9. Nutritional value per serving, omitting rice and assuming complete consumption of sauce.

NUTRITION

Calories: 465cal (23%)Carbohydrates: 22g (7%)Protein: 32g (64%)Fat: 28g (43%)Saturated Fat: 14g (88%)Cholesterol: 143mg (48%)Sodium: 974mg (42%)Potassium: 446mg (13%)Fiber: 1g (4%)Sugar: 10g (11%)Vitamin A: 110IU (2%)Vitamin C: 1mg (1%)Calcium: 26mg (3%)Iron: 2mg (11%)

74. LEMON PEPPER CHICKEN

PREP TIME: 15 MINS

TOTAL TIME: 45 MINS

INGREDIENTS

- 1/2 c. all-purpose flour
- 1 tbsp. lemon pepper seasoning
- 1 tsp. kosher salt
- 2 lemons, divided
- 1 lb. boneless skinless chicken breasts, halved
- 2 tbsp. extra-virgin olive oil
- 1/2 c. Chicken broth
- 2 tbsp. butter
- 2 cloves garlic, minced
- Freshly chopped parsley, for garnish

DIRECTIONS

Preheat the oven to 400 degrees Fahrenheit. mix flour, lemon pepper, salt, and 1 lemon zest in a medium mixing basin. Coat the chicken breasts in the flour blender until they are completely covered. The remaining lemon should be sliced into thin rounds. Warm oil in a big ovenproof skillet over medium-high heat. Cook, in a single layer, until golden brown on the bottom, about 5 minutes, then turn the chicken breasts.

Add the stock, butter, garlic, and lemon slices to the pan and bake for 5 minutes, or until the chicken is cooked through and the sauce has reduced somewhat.

Garnish with parsley and a dollop of sauce on top of the chicken.

FOR STOVETOP

mix flour, lemon pepper, salt, and 1 lemon zest in a medium mixing basin. Coat the chicken breasts in the flour mixture until they are completely covered. The remaining lemon should be sliced into thin rounds.

Warm oil in a big ovenproof skillet over medium-high hot. Make, in a single layer, before golden brown on the bottom, about 5 minutes, then turn the chicken breasts.

Add the stock, butter, garlic, and lemon slices to the skillet and simmer for 3 minutes, or until the chicken is cooked through and the sauce has reduced somewhat.

Garnish with parsley and a dollop of sauce on top of the chicken.

75. KETO FRIED CHICKEN

PREP TIME: 15 MINS

TOTAL TIME:1 HOUR 15 MINS

INGREDIENTS

- 6 bone-in, skin-on chicken breasts
- Kosher salt
- Freshly ground black pepper
- 2 big eggs
- 1/2 c. heavy cream
- 3/4 c. almond flour
- 1 1/2 c. finely crushed pork rinds
- 1/2 c. freshly grated Parmesan
- 1 tsp. garlic powder
- 1/2 tsp. paprika

FOR THE SPICY MAYO

- 1/2 c. mayonnaise
- 1 1/2 tsp. hot sauce

DIRECTIONS

Warm the oven to 400° Fand prepare a large baking sheet with parchment paper. Season the chicken with salt and pepper after patting it dry with paper towels.

Whisk together the eggs and heavy cream in a shallow bowl. mix almond flour, pork rinds, Parmesan, garlic powder, and paprika in a small bowl. Salt & pepper as need.

Dip each chicken piece in the egg blender, then in the almond flour mixture, pressing to coat. Place the chicken on the baking sheet that has been prepared.

Bake for 45 minutes, or before the chicken is golden brown and the internal temperature reaches 165°.

Make the dipping sauce in the meantime: mix mayonnaise and spicy sauce in a medium mixing basin. Depending on your chosen degree of spiciness, add additional hot sauce.

Serve the chicken with the dipping sauce while it's still warm.

76. AIR FRYER TURKEY BREAST

PREP TIME:5 mins

COOK TIME:55 mins

TOTAL TIME:1 hr

INGREDIENTS

- 4 pound turkey breast, on the bone with skin (ribs removed)
- 1 tbspolive oil
- 2 tsp kosher
- 1/2 tbspdry turkey or poultry seasoning, I used Bell's which has not salt

INSTRUCTIONS

1 tbspoil, rubbed all over the turkey breast Rub the remaining half tbspof oil over the skin side after coating both sides with salt and turkey spice.

Preheat the air fryer to 350°F and cook the skin side down for 20 minutes. Turn over and cook for another 30 to 40 minutes, depending on the size of your breast, until the internal temperature reaches 160°F using an instant-read thermometer. Allow 10 minutes for resting before cutting.

NOTES

The smart points will be 0 without the skin.

Nutrition

Serving: 4ounces, Calories: 226kcal, Protein: 32.5g, Fat: 10g, Saturated Fat: 2.5g, Cholesterol: 84mg, Sodium: 296mg Blue Smart Points:4 Green Smart Points:5 Purple Smart Points:5 Points +:4

77. KETO FRIED CHICKEN

YIELDS:6 - 8 SERVINGS

PREP TIME:0 HOURS 15 MINS

TOTAL TIME:1 HOUR 15 MINS

INGREDIENTS
FOR THE CHICKEN

- 6 bone-in, skin-on chicken breasts
- Kosher salt
- Freshly ground black pepper
- 2 big eggs
- 1/2 c. heavy cream
- 3/4 c. almond flour
- 1 1/2 c. finely crushed pork rinds
- 1/2 c. freshly grated Parmesan
- 1 tsp. garlic powder
- 1/2 tsp. paprika

FOR THE SPICY MAYO

- 1/2 c. mayonnaise
- 1 1/2 tsp. hot sauce

DIRECTIONS

Warm the oven to 400° Fand prepare a large baking sheet with parchment paper. Season the chicken with salt and pepper after patting it dry with paper towels.

Whisk together the eggs and heavy cream in a shallow bowl. mix almond flour, pork rinds, Parmesan, garlic powder, and paprika in a small bowl. Salt & pepper as need.

Dip each chicken piece in the egg blender, then in the almond flour mixture, pressing to coat. Place the chicken on the baking sheet that has been prepared.

Bake for 45 minutes, or before the chicken is golden brown and the internal temperature reaches 165°.

Make the dipping sauce in the meantime: mix mayonnaise and spicy sauce in a medium mixing basin. Depending on your chosen degree of spiciness, add additional hot sauce.

Serve the chicken with the dipping sauce while it's still warm.

78. CREAMY CAJUN CHICKEN

PREP TIME:10 mins

COOK TIME:20 mins

TOTAL TIME:30 mins

INGREDIENTS

- 2 large chicken breasts sliced in half lengthwise
- Salt & pepper as need
- 1/4 tsp garlic powder
- 1/2 tsp + 1 tbspCajun seasoning (use a no or low salt variety)
- Flour for dredging
- 2 tbsp butter
- 1 tbspolive oil
- 3 cloves garlic minced
- 1/4 cups ofun-dried tomatoes
- 1/4 cup ofchicken broth
- 1 cup ofheavy/whipping cream
- 1/2 cup offreshly grated parmesan cheese

INSTRUCTIONS

Make four thinner cutlets by halving the chicken lengthwise. Add salt, pepper, garlic powder, and 1/2 tsp of Cajun spice as need. Using flour, coat them.

In a pan over medium-high heat, melt the butter and oil. Add the chicken once the pan is heated. Cook for 4-5 minutes per side, or until golden brown. Add the lid from the pan and place it on a plate.

Toss in the sun-dried tomatoes, garlic, and chicken stock to the pan. Allow it to bubble for around 30 seconds.

Reduce the heat to medium-low and add the cream and 1 tbspof Cajun spice.

Add the chicken to the skillet and continue cooking for another 5 minutes, or until the sauce has thickened slightly and the chicken is cooked through. Top with a sprinkling of parmesan Parmesan (or stir it into the sauce). Season with salt and pepper as need and serve right away.

NOTES

Because this recipe contains a lot of Cajun seasoning, I strongly advise you to choose one that isn't salty. Otherwise, the meal will be far too salty. Tony Chachere's No Salt Creole Seasoning was utilized.

I used oil-packed sun-dried tomatoes that I drained before putting in the pan.

If you have smaller chicken breasts, you may cook them whole, but they'll take a little longer to cook.

NUTRITION

Calories: 499kcal,Carbohydrates: 9g,Protein: 32g,Fat: 38g,Saturated Fat: 21g,Trans Fat: 1g,Cholesterol: 180mg,Sodium: 466mg,Potassium: 749mg,Fiber: 1g,Sugar: 3g,Vitamin A: 1437IU,Vitamin C: 6mg,Calcium: 198mg,Iron: 1mg.

79. CHICKEN PAPRIKA

Preparation time: 30 mins

Cooking time: 1 to 2 hours

Ingredients

- 1 large chicken, jointed (or use 2 large chicken legs and 2 breasts, halved)
- salt
- 2 tbsp olive oil
- knob butter
- 1 onion, chopped
- 2-3 cloves garlic, chopped
- 2 tbsp sweet paprika, or 1 tbsp each sweet and hot paprika
- 1 tbsp flour
- 285ml/½pint chicken stock
- 3 tbsp chopped fresh flatleaf parsley
- 2 red peppers, seeds take and cut into 1cm/0.5in strips
- 4 large ripe tomatoes, roughly chopped
- 250ml/8fl oz soured cream

INSTRUCTIONS

Season the chicken with salt. In a big heavy-bottomed skillet, heat the oil and butter and brown the chicken all over for a few minutes. Pull the chicken out of the plate and set it aside.

Add the onions and garlic to the same pan and cook for about 5 minutes. Stir in the paprika, then the flour until well mixed, being careful not to burn it.

Pour in the stock and give it a good swirl. Back the chicken to the pan, adding a small more stock if the mixture appears to be too dry. Bring to a boil with half of the parsley. Reduce the heat to low and cook the red pepper strips for 10 minutes. Stir in the tomatoes and cook for 1 hour on low heat.

Take the pan from the heat after the chicken is done. mix the sour cream and the remaining parsley in a mixing bowl. Season as need and serve.

80. KOREAN FRIED CHICKEN

PREP TIME: 15 MINS

TOTAL TIME:1 HOUR 0 MINS

INGREDIENTS

- Vegetable oil
- 1 tsp. kosher salt
- 1/2 tsp. freshly ground black pepper
- 1/2 tsp. baking powder
- 1/2 tsp. garlic powder
- 2 lb. chicken wings
- 1 tbsp. freshly grated ginger
- 1/2 c. cornstarch

FOR SAUCE

- 3 tbsp. butter
- 5 small dried red chilis, sliced
- 1 tbsp. freshly minced ginger
- 3 cloves garlic, minced
- 1/4 c. gochujang
- 2 tbsp. ketchup
- 1 tbsp. rice vinegar
- 1 tbsp. low-sodium soy sauce
- 1/4 c. honey
- 2 tbsp. packed brown sugar

FOR GARNISH

- 1/2 c. cocktail peanuts
- 1 tbsp. sesame seeds
- 1 green onion, sliced

DIRECTIONS

To make the wings, follow these steps: Heat 4 to 6 cups of vegetable oil to 275° in a deep saucepan over medium-high heat. Paper towels should be used to line a large plate or baking sheet. mix salt, pepper, baking powder, and garlic powder in a small basin.

Dry the wings using paper towels before rubbing them with grated ginger and seasoning them with the salt mixture. Toss wings with cornstarch in a large mixing basin and crush to compact coating onto each wing.

Carefully place wings in the oil and fried until the skin is lightly crisped and brown, approximately 15 to 18 minutes, turning with tongs as needed. Remove the wings from the oil and place them on a plate that has been prepared. Allow it cool for a few minutes.

Preheat the frying oil to 400 degrees. Return the wings to the saucepan and cook for another 7 to 8 minutes, or until the skin is crisp and crispy. Place the wings in a large mixing bowl after taking them from the oil.

To make the sauce, mix the butter, dried chilis, ginger, and garlic in a medium saucepan over medium-low heat and simmer for 2 minutes, or until aromatic. Cook until gochujang, ketchup, vinegar, and soy sauce have bubbled up. Cook, stirring constantly, until the honey and brown sugar have dissolved and the sauce has thickened somewhat.

Toss the wings in the sauce until they are uniformly covered. Toss in the peanuts to mix.

Before serving, sprinkle with sesame seeds and green onion.

81. SWEET AND SOUR CHICKEN

Prep Time: 15 minutes

Cook Time: 10 minutes

Total Time: 25 minutes

Ingredients

- 1 1/2 lbs chicken breasts
- 1/2 cup ofcornstarch
- 2 eggs beaten
- 1/4 cup offlour
- canola oil for frying
- 1 cup ofpineapple chunks
- 1 red bell pepper
- 1 green bell pepper
- 1/2 yellow onion
- 1/2 cups ofugar
- 1/4 cup ofbrown sugar
- 1/2 cup ofapple cider vinegar
- 1/3 cup ofketchup
- 4 tsp reduced sodium soy sauce
- 2 cloves garlic minced

Instructions

In a little bowl, blend the sugar, brown sugar, apple cider vinegar, ketchup, soy sauce, and garlic to make the sauce.

Fill a dutch oven halfway with canola oil or sizzling pan to reach up about an inch to an inch and a half from the bottom.

Warm the oil over medium-high to high hot for approximately 2-3 minutes, just until the chicken is cooked and browned.

Fill a big ziplock bag halfway with cornstarch.

Shake the chicken pieces in the big ziplock bag until they are well covered.

Before putting the pieces in the heated oil, dip them in the egg, then the flour.

Make for 2-3 minutes, or before the chicken is cooked through and crispy.

Place on a cookie sheet to cool (no paper towels!). Continue to cook the chicken pieces before they're all done.

Remove everything except a tbspof the oil from the pan once it's finished cooking.

Cook for 1-2 minutes, until the bell peppers, onion, and pineapple are crisp-tender.

Bake the sauce to the pan and swirl to coat the pieces, then simmer for 30 seconds to reheat the garlic.

Stir in the chicken pieces until the sauce has thickened and is boiling.

Serve immediately with sesame seeds or green onions as toppings.

Nutrition

Yield: 4 , Amount per serving: 602 calories, Calories: 602g, Carbohydrates: 92g, Protein: 41g, Fat: 6g, Saturated Fat: 1g, Cholesterol: 190mg, Sodium: 588mg, Potassium: 1082mg, Fiber: 3g, Sugar: 65g, Vitamin A: 1385g, Vitamin C: 79.5g, Calcium: 67g, Iron: 2.4g

82. CHICKEN TIKKA MASALA

PREP:15 MINS

COOK:30 MINS

TOTAL:45 MINS

INGREDIENTS

For the chicken marinade:

- 28 oz boneless and skinless chicken thighs
- 1 cup ofplain yogurt
- 1 1/2 tbsp minced garlic
- 1 tbspginger
- 2 tsp garam masala
- 1 tsp turmeric
- 1 tsp ground cumin
- 1 tsp Kashmiri chili (or 1/2 tsp ground red chili powder)
- 1 tsp of salt

For the sauce:

- 2 tbsp of vegetable/canola oil
- 2 tbsp butter
- 2 small onions finely diced
- 1 1/2 tbsp garlic finely grated
- 1 tbspginger finely grated
- 1 1/2 tsp garam masala
- 1 1/2 tsp ground cumin
- 1 tsp turmeric powder

- 1 tsp ground coriander
- 14 oz (400g) tomato puree (tomato sauce/Passata)
- 1 tsp Kashmiri chili (optional for colour and flavour)
- 1 tsp ground red chili powder
- 1 tsp salt
- 1 1/4 cups of heavy or thickened cream (use evaporated milk for lower calories)
- 1 tsp brown sugar
- 1/4 cup of water if needed
- 4 tbsp coriander leaves or cilantro to give as a decoration

INSTRUCTIONS

mix the chicken with all of the ingredients for the chicken marinade in a mixing bowl; set aside for 10 minutes to an hour to marinate (or overnight if time allows).

In a large skillet or saucepan, heat the oil over medium-high heat. When the pan is hot, add the chicken pieces in two or three batches, being careful not to crowd the pan. Make for just 3 minutes on each side until golden. Remove from oven and keep warm. (The chicken will finish cooking in the sauce.)

In the same pan, melt the butter. Cook until the onions are soft (approximately 3 minutes), scraping away any browned pieces from the bottom of the pan.

Sauté for 1 minute, or until garlic and ginger are aromatic, then add garam masala, cumin, turmeric, and coriander. Cook for about 20 seconds, stirring periodically, until aromatic.

mix the tomato puree, chili powders, and salt in a mixing bowl. Allow sauce to boil for 10-15 minutes, stirring periodically, until it thickens and turns a rich brown red color.

In a big mixing bowl, blend the cream and sugar. Return the chicken to the pan with its juices and simmer for another 8-10 minutes, or until the chicken is cooked through and the sauce is rich and boiling. If the sauce has to be thinned, add the water.

Serve with hot garlic butter rice and fresh handmade Naan bread, garnished with cilantro (coriander).

NUTRITION

Cals: 580kcal, Dietary carbohydrate: 17g, Starch: 36g, Chubby: 41g,Saturated Fat: 19g, Blood sugar: 250mg, Sodium: 1601mg, Potassium: 973mg, Fiber: 3g, Sugar: 8g, Vitamin A: 1895IU, Vitamin C: 19.5mg, Calcium: 171mg, Iron: 4.1mg, Vitamin A: 1895IU, Vitamin C: 19.5

83. HERB-ROASTED TURKEY BREAST

Prep: 25 min

Inactive: 15 min

Cook: 2 hr

Total: 2 hr 40 min

Ingredients

- 1 whole bone-in turkey breast
- 1 tbspminced garlic (3 cloves
- 2 tsp dry mustard

- 1 tbsp chopped fresh rosemary leave
- 1 tbsp chopped fresh sage leaves
- 1 tsp chopped fresh thyme leaves
- 2 tsp kosher salt
- 1 tsp freshly ground black pepper
- 2 tbsp good olive oil
- 2 tbsp freshly squeezed lemon juice
- 1 cup of dry white wine

Directions

Preheat oven to 325 degrees Fahrenheit. Arrange your turkey breast skin side up on a shelf in a grill pan.

To produce a paste, mix together the garlic, mustard, herbs, salt, pepper, olive oil, and lemon juice in a small bowl. With your fingers, carefully loosen the skin from the flesh and smear half of the mixture directly on the meat. Massage the leftover paste to the skin in an equal layer. Pour the wine into the roasting pan's bottom.

Roast the turkey for 1 3/4 to 2 hours, or until the skin is golden brown and an instant-read thermometer reads 165 degrees Fahrenheit.

When placed into the thickest and meatiest regions of the breast, a read thermometer detects 165 degrees F. (I do tests in a variety of locations.) Aluminum foil should be used to cover the chest loosely if the skin is over-browning. When the turkey is done, cover it with foil and set it aside to rest for 15 minutes at room temperature. Slice the turkey and serve with the pan juices spooned over it.

84. MAPLE ROAST TURKEY

Prep:1 hr

Cook:3 hrs 30 mins

Additional:2 hrs

Total:6 hrs 30 mins

Ingredients

- 2 cups of apple cider
- ⅓ cup ofreal maple syrup
- 2 ½ tbsp chopped fresh thyme
- 2 tbsp chopped fresh marjora
- 1 ½ tsp grated lemon zest
- ¾ cup ofbutter, softened
- salt and pepper to tast
- 1 (12 pound) whole turkey, neck and giblets reserved
- 2 cups of chopped onion
- 1 ½ cups of chopped celery
- 1 ½ cups of chopped carrots
- 3 cups of chicken brot
- ¼ cup ofall-purpose flour
- 1 bay leaf
- ½ cup ofapple brandy

Instructions

In a saucepan, mix apple cider and maple syrup and bring to a boil over medium-high heat.Make before the liquid has been reduced to 1/2 cup, then remove the pan from the heat. 1

tbspthyme, 1 tbspmarjoram, and 1 tbsplemon zest Season with salt and pepper after stirring in the butter until it has melted. Cover and chill until ready to serve. Warm the oven to 375 degrees Fahrenheit. Place the oven rack in the smallest third of the oven.

Place the turkey in a roasting pan on a rack. 1/4 cup ofmaple butter is set aside for gravy, and the remaining maple butter is rubbed under the skin of the turkey's breast and all over the exterior. Surround the turkey with onion, celery, carrots, turkey neck, and giblets. 1 tbspthyme, 1 tbspmarjoram, 1 tbspthyme, 1 tbspmarjoram, 1 tbspthyme, 1 tbspmarjoram, Fill the pan with 2 cups ofbroth.

In a preheated oven, roast the turkey for 30 minutes.Warm the oven to 350 degrees Fahrenheit . Cover the entire turkey with foil. Continue to grill for another 2 1/2 hours, or until a meat thermometer inserted into the thickest portion of the thigh reads 180°F (85 degrees C). Place the turkey on a plate and set aside for 30 minutes. Remove any extra fat from the pan juices and strain them into a large measuring cup. To make 3 cups ofchicken broth, add enough chicken stock to the pan juices. Fill a pot halfway with liquid and bring to a boil. 1/4 cup ofmaple butter and 1/3 cup offlour, mixd in a small bowl until smooth. Whisk together all the flour and butter in a different basin. Add the bay leaf and the rest of the thyme. Cook, stirring periodically, until the sauce has reduced to a sauce consistency, about 10 minutes. If desired, add apple brandy. As need, season with salt and pepper.

Nutrition

Per Serving: 872 calories; protein 91.6g; carbohydrates 21.2g; fat 43.1g; cholesterol 295mg; sodium 330.9mg.

85. CARIBBEAN CHICKEN

Total: 8 hr 30 min

Prep: 10 min

Inactive: 8 hr

Cook: 20 min

Ingredients

- 1 tsp allspice
- 1/4 cup ofred onion, chopped
- 1/2 cup ofgreen onions, chopped
- 2 tbsp extra-virgin olive oil
- 1/4 cup oforange juice, fresh
- 1 tbsplime zest
- 2 tbsp soy sauce
- 2 tbsp freshly chopped thyme leaves
- 2 tbsp jalapeno, seeded, diced
- 2 tsp freshly grated or chopped ginger
- 1 clove garlic
- Salt and pepper
- 4 chicken breasts, bone and skin on
- Lime wedges

Directions

Sautee all items except for the chicken in a food processor. In a re-sealable plastic bag, mix the marinade and the chicken, stir completely, and refrigerate for 4 to 8 hours.

Preheat the oven to 350 degrees Fahrenheit.

Preheat the grill to high, then remove the chicken from the marinade and set it on the grill. Roast for 3 to 4 minutes on each side, then transfer to a pan and finish in the oven for 15 minutes.

Serve with a lime wedge squeezed over each piece of chicken.

86. CHICKEN PICCATA

Total: 40 min

Prep: 15 min

Cook: 25 min

Ingredients

- 2 skinless and boneless chicken breasts, butterflied and then cut in half
- Sea salt and freshly ground black pepper
- All-purpose flour, for dredging
- 6 tbsp unsalted butter
- 5 tbsp extra-virgin olive oil
- 1/3 cup offresh lemon juice
- 1/2 cup ofchicken stock
- 1/4 cup ofbrined capers, rinsed
- 1/3 cup offresh parsley, chopped

Directions

Period the chicken with salt and pepper before serving. Using flour, dredge the chicken and shake off the excess.

Melt 2 tbsp butter and 3 tbsp olive oil in a large pan over medium high heat. Add 2 pieces of chicken and fry for 3 minutes after the butter and oil have started to sizzle.Make for 3 minutes on the opposite side when the chicken has browned. Remove from the pan and place on a platter. 2 tbsp butter, 2 tbsp olive oil, 2 tbsp butter, 2 tbsp olive oil, 2 tbsp olive oil, 2 tbsp olive oil, 2 tbsp olive oil When the butter and oil have begun to sizzle, add the remaining two pieces of chicken and brown on same parties in the same manner. Remove the pan from the heat and place the chicken on a platter.

Add the lemon juice, stock, and capers to the pan. Return to the burner and bring to a boil, scraping up any brown pieces that have accumulated in the pan for added flavor. Seasoning should be checked. Transfer the chicken to the pan in its entirety and continue to cook for another 5 minutes. Place the chicken on a serving platter. Whisk the remaining 2 tbsp butter into the sauce quickly. Pour the sauce over the chicken and sprinkle the parsley on top.

87. THAI CHICKEN

Prep:20 mins

Cook:30 mins

Total:50 mins

Ingredients

- 1 cups ofoy sauce
- 8 cloves garlic, minced
- 1 tbspminced fresh ginger root
- 2 tbsp hot pepper sauce
- 2 pounds skinless chicken thighs
- 1 tbspsesame oil
- 1 tbspbrown sugar
- 1 onion, sliced
- ½ cup ofwater
- 4 tbsp crunchy peanut butter
- 2 tbsp green onions, chopped

Instructions

mix the soy sauce, garlic, ginger, and hot pepper sauce in a large mixing basin. Mix thoroughly, then add the chicken to the bowl, turning to coat evenly. Refrigerate for at least one hour after covering and marinating. In a Dutch oven, heat the sesame oil over medium high heat. Stir in the brown sugar until it is completely dissolved. Cook for 5 minutes after adding the onion. Add the chicken pieces and make for 5 minutes, rotating once to ensure uniform browning. Bring the marinade to a boil, then add the water. Reduce to a low heat and cook for 15 to 20 minutes. Stir in the peanut butter and continue to cook for another 10 minutes.Arrange the chickens on a baking tray with the sauce and chives on top.

Nutrition

Per Serving: 466 calories; protein 53.4g; carbohydrates 16.8g; fat 20.5g; cholesterol 188.4mg; sodium 3930.3mg.

88. SPICY DRY-RUBBED CHICKEN WINGS RECIPE

Prep: 5 mins

Cook: 50 mins

Ready in: 55 mins

Ingredients

- 2 lbs

Spicy Dry Rub Recipe

- 2 tbsp Smoked Paprika
- 3 tsp Cayenne Pepper, optional
- 2 tsp Chili Powder
- 1 tbsp Black Pepper
- 1.5 tbsp Garlic Powder
- 2 tsp Onion Powder

- 1.5 tbsp Natural Ancient Sea Salt
- 1.5 tsp Italian Seasoning
- 1.5 tsp dried thyme

Instructions

To marinate the chicken wings, place them in a ziploc bag with 1/4 cup of the spicy dry rub. The remaining can be kept in a mason jar.

Shake the bag to evenly coat the chicken in the mixture.

Refrigerate for at least four hours, preferably overnight.

Before you start cooking:

Add the lid from of the fridge and set it aside to come to room temperature (30 minutes). Preheat the oven to 400 degrees Fahrenheit.

For the oven, prepare the following:

Using parchment paper, line a cookie sheet. Arrange the chicken wings on the paper in an equal pattern.

Cook each side for 20-25 minutes.

If you're a Ninja Foodi, here's what you should do.

In the air fryer basket, place the chicken wings.

Cook each side for 15 minutes.

Nutrition

Calories: 206kcal | Carbohydrates: 5g | Protein: 16g | Fat: 14g | Saturated Fat: 4g | Cholesterol: 63mg | Sodium: 1819mg | Potassium: 264mg | Fiber: 2g | Sugar: 1g | Vitamin A: 1901IU | Vitamin C: 1mg | Calcium: 37mg | Iron: 2m

89. PECAN CRUSTED CHICKEN

PREP:25 mins

COOK:20 mins

TOTAL:50 mins

Ingredients
FOR THE PECAN CRUSTED CHICKEN:

- 2 large eggs
- 1 cup ofpecan halves
- 1/2 cup ofPanko bread crumbs
- 1 tsp dried basil
- 1/2 tsp kosher salt
- 1/4 tsp coarse black pepper
- 4 little boneless, skinless chicken breasts about 6 ounces each
- 2 tbsp extra virgin olive oil

FOR THE HONEY MUSTARD DIPPING SAUCE:

- 1 cup ofnonfat plain Greek yogurt

- 2 tbsp Dijon mustard
- 1 ½ tbsp grainy brown mustard or an additional tbsp of Dijon
- 1 tbsp honey + additional as need
- ¼ tsp kosher salt
- Pinch cayenne pepper

Instructions

Warm the oven to 400 degrees Fahrenheit with a rack in the center. Using parchment paper or a silicone baking mat, line a large baking sheet.

In a broad, shallow bowl or pie plate, lightly beat the eggs and leave aside.

Pulse the nuts in a food processor until fine crumbs form (don't over-process or they'll turn into pecan butter). Fill a big, strong ziptop bag halfway with the mixture.

Nuts, crushed in a food processor

Add the breadcrumbs, basil, salt, and pepper to the bag. Seal the top and give it a good shake to mix everything.

Nuts smashed in a bag

Cover the chicken with a big sheet of plastic wrap and place it on a chopping board. Pound the chicken breasts to a uniform thickness using a meat tenderizer, rolling pin, or your fist. They don't have to be extremely thin; simply flatten the centre to ensure that the chicken bakes evenly.

The pounding of chicken breasts

Working with one chicken breast at a time, dip it in the egg wash, then place it in the ziptop bag with the pecan mixture and shake it to coat it. Place the chicken on the prepared roasting sheet and gently press the pecan mixture to adhere to it. Rep with the rest of the chicken breasts.

Meat that has been dipped in an egg wash

Drizzle the olive oil over the chicken and serve. Bake for 15 to 20 minutes, or until an instant read thermometer reads 160 to 165 degrees F. Remove to a platter and set aside for 5 minutes to cool. Cooking chicken to 165 degrees F is considered done, but I prefer to remove mine a few degrees earlier and allow the carryover cooking do the job (this ensures the chicken breast is juicy and does not overcook).

4 chicken breasts with honey pecan crust
Prepare the sauce while the chicken bakes: mix the Greek yogurt, both mustards, honey, salt, and cayenne in a small mixing bowl. Season as need and adjust seasoning as needed.
In a bowl, the sauce components are being mixed.
Serve the pecan crusted chicken with the dipping sauce while it's still hot.
Chicken with a pecan crust and honey mustard sauce

Notes

TO STORE: Keep the chicken refrigerated for up to 3 days in an airtight container.
Heat it up: Finn wolfhard leftovers in the oven at 350°F for a few minutes on a baking sheet.
TO FREEZE: Freeze chicken for up to 3 months in an airtight freezer-safe storage container. Allow to defrost in the refrigerator overnight before reheating.

A strawberry and goat cheese topping was used in an early version of this recipe. We've subsequently learned to favor the honey mustard dip's simplicity. If you want to try this version, follow these steps: 1 tsp olive oil, 12 cups of strawberries, 2 tbsp balsamic vinegar, 14 tsp dried basil, and 18 tsp kosher salt in a small saucepan Cook, stirring periodically, until the sauce has thickened, about 10 minutes. Strawberry sauce and crumbled goat cheese are served on top of roasted chicken.

Nutrition

CALORIES: 489kcal,CARBOHYDRATES: 9g,PROTEIN: 42g,FAT: 32g,SATURATED FAT: 4g,TRANS FAT: 1g,CHOLESTEROL: 191mg,POTASSIUM: 784mg,FIBER: 3g,SUGAR: 2g,VITAMIN A: 186IU,VITAMIN C: 2mg,CALCIUM: 58mg,IRON: 2mg.

90. CHICKEN MEATBALLS

Prep Time 10 minutes

Cook Time 20 minutes

Total Time 30 minutes

INGREDIENTS

- 2 pounds ground chicken 96% lean
- 1 egg
- 1 cup ofpanko breadcrumbs
- 1/2 cup ofgrated parmesan cheese
- 2 tbsp olive oil
- 1 tsp minced garlic
- 1 tsp salt
- 1/2 tsp pepper
- 1 tsp dried Italian seasoning
- cooking spray
- 1 tbspchopped parsley

INSTRUCTIONS

Preheat oven to 400 degrees Fahrenheit. Warm a sheet pan by lining it with foil and spraying it with cooking spray.

In a mixing bowl, mix the ground chicken, eggs, breadcrumbs, parmesan cheese, olive oil, garlic, salt, and pepper, as well as the Italian seasoning. Mix until everything is well mixed.

Roll the meatballs into 1 inch balls and arrange them in a single layer on the baking sheet.

Bake for 20 minutes, or before meatballs are cooked through and browned. Serve with a parsley garnish.

NUTRITION

Calories: 310kcal | Carbohydrates: 6g | Protein: 29g | Fat: 19g | Saturated Fat: 5g | Cholesterol: 185mg | Sodium: 554mg | Potassium: 824mg | Fiber: 1g | Sugar: 1g | Vitamin A: 80IU | Vitamin C: 0.2mg | Calcium: 36mg | Iron: 2mg.

91. EASY CHICKEN TACOS

prep time: 15 MINUTES

cook time: 15 MINUTES

total time: 30 MINUTES

INGREDIENTS:

- 2 tsp chili powder
- 1 tsp ground cumin
- 1 tsp smoked paprika
- 1 tsp dried oregano
- 1/2 tsp garlic powder
- Kosher sodium chloride and freshly ground black pepper, as need
- 1 1/2 pounds boneless, skinless chicken thighs
- 1 tbsp canola oil
- 12 mini flour tortillas, warmed
- 1 cup of pico de gallo, homemade or store-bought
- 1 avocado, halved, peeled, seeded and diced
- 1/2 cup of chopped fresh cilantro leaves
- 1 lime, cut into wedges

DIRECTIONS:

mix chili powder, cumin, paprika, oregano, garlic powder, 1 tsp salt, and 1/2 tsp pepper in a small mixing bowl. Chili powder mixture is used to season the chicken.

In a large skillet, heat the canola oil over medium-high heat. Working in batches, place the chicken in a single layer in the skillet and fry until golden brown and cooked through, about 4-5 minutes each side, or until an internal temperature of 165 degrees F is reached. Allow it cool completely before slicing into bite-size pieces.

Serve the chicken with pico de gallo, avocado, cilantro, and lime on tortillas.

92. AIR FRYER FRIED CHICKEN KFC COPYCAT

PREP TIME:12 hours

COOK TIME:26 minutes

TOTAL TIME:12 hours 26 minutes

Ingredients

- 10 chicken drumsticks or thighs
- 1 cup ofButtermilk
- 2 eggs
- 2 cups of flour
- 2/3 tsp salt
- Half tsp thyme
- 1/2 tsp basil
- 1/3 tsp oregano
- 1 tsp celery salt

- Tsp black pepper
- One tsp dried mustard
- 4 tsp paprika
- 2 tsp garlic salt
- 1 tsp ground ginger
- 3 tsp white pepper

Instructions

Before beginning this recipe, soak the chicken legs in buttermilk for up to 24 hours.

Beat the eggs in one plate and the milk in the other, whisk together the flour and spices. The spices should be well mixed into the flour, and the eggs should be lightly beaten.

Place a baking sheet on top of an oven-safe cooling rack.

Remove the chicken from the buttermilk one piece at a time.

Dredge each chicken leg in flour, then in eggs, and then back in flour. Place the coated drumstick on a cooling rack and continue with the rest of the chicken.

Preheat the Air Fryer at 390 degrees.

To protect the chicken from adhering to the bottom of the air fryer, place a Parchment circle in the bottom.

In a Ninja Foodie or Air Fryer, arrange the chicken in a single layer so the pieces don't touch.

Air Preheat the oven to 350°F and fry for 13 minutes. Toss it over. You may spray with olive oil if there are any dry places where the flour is visible. Continue to fry for another 13 minutes. Make sure the interior temperature is 165 degrees. If not, cook for an additional 5 minutes at a time until done.

Enjoy!

Directions for Deep Fried and Oven Fried Chicken:

6+ cups of oil (peanut or vegetable) of choice (for deep frying version)

Preheat the oven to 300 degrees Fahrenheit.
Before beginning this recipe, soak the chicken legs in buttermilk for up to 24 hours.
In one bowl, crack the eggs; in another, mix the flour and spices. The spices should be well mixed into the flour, and the eggs should be lightly beaten.
Overtop a baking sheet with an oven-safe cooling rack; this will serve two roles during the procedure.
Remove the chicken from the buttermilk one piece at a time.
Dredge each chicken leg in flour, then in eggs, and then back in flour. Place the coated drumstick on a cooling rack and continue with the rest of the chicken. In a big dutch oven or stockpot, warm the oil over medium-high heat. (Alternatively, a deep fryer can be used.) Fry the chicken legs in groups of three for 2-4 minutes, or until golden brown.
Place the chicken on a cooling rack and continue with the rest of the chicken.
If you're going to bake anything in the oven,
Follow the procedures, except instead of frying in oil, bake in the oven.
Bake for 35-45 minutes, or until a thermometer inserted in the center registers 165 degrees Fahrenheit.

Nutrition

Amount Per Serving: CALORIES: 1063TOTAL FAT: 39gSATURATED FAT: 11gTRANS FAT: 0gUNSATURATED FAT: 24gCHOLESTEROL: 568mgSODIUM: 2518mgCARBOHYDRATES: 73gFIBER: 4gSUGAR: 5gPROTEIN: 100g.

93. OREGANO CHICKEN

Ingredients

- ¼ cup of butter, melted
- ¼ cup of lemon juice
- 2 tbsp Worcestershire sauce
- 2 tbsp soy sauce
- 2 tsp dried oregano
- 1 tsp garlic powder
- 6 skinless, boneless chicken breast halves

Instructions

Warm the oven to 375 degrees Fahrenheit. Melt the butter or margarine and blend it with the lemon juice, Worcestershire sauce, soy sauce, oregano, and garlic powder. Mix thoroughly. Place the chicken in a 7x11 inch baking dish that hasn't been oiled. Over the chicken, pour the butter/oregano mixture. Bake for 15 minutes in a preheated oven. Brush the chicken with the juices. Make for another 15 minutes at 350°F. Transfer the chicken to a serving plate and, if preferred, spoon the pan drippings over hot cooked rice.

Nutrition

Per Serving: 180 calories; protein 23.9g; carbohydrates 2.6g; fat 7.9g; cholesterol 76.1mg; sodium 418mg.

94. TURKEY BRINE

Prep: 5 mins

Cook: 15 mins

Additional: 8 hrs

Total: 8 hrs 20 mins

Ingredients

- 1 gallon vegetable broth
- 1 cups ofea salt
- 1 tbsp crushed dried rosemary
- 1 tbsp dried sage
- 1 tbsp dried thyme
- 1 tbsp dried savory
- 1 gallon ice water

Instructions

mix the vegetable broth, sea salt, rosemary, sage, thyme, and savory in a large stock pot. Bring to a boil, stirring constantly to ensure that the salt is completely dissolved. Allow to cool to room temperature after withdrawing from the heat. Pour the broth mixture into a clean 5 gallon bucket once it has cooled. Add the ice water and mix well.

Your turkey should be washed and dried. Check to see if the insides have been removed. Place the turkey in the brine, breast down. Ascertain that the cavity is completely filled. Refrigerate the bucket for at least one night.

Carefully drain the extra brine from the turkey and pat it dry. Excess brine should be discarded.

Cook the turkey according to your preferences, saving the drippings for gravy. Remember that brined turkeys cook 20 to 30 minutes faster, so keep an eye on the thermometer.

Nutrition

Per Serving: 3 calories; protein 0.1g; carbohydrates 0.6g; fat 0.1g; cholesterol 0mg; sodium 5640.3mg.

95. BLACKENED CHICKEN

Prep: 10 mins

Cook: 10 mins

Total: 20 mins

Ingredients

- ½ tsp paprika
- ⅛ tsp salt
- ¼ tsp cayenne pepper
- ¼ tsp ground cumin
- ¼ tsp dried thyme
- ⅛ tsp ground white pepper
- ⅛ tsp onion powder
- 2 skinless, boneless chicken breast halves

Instructions

Warm the oven to 350 degrees Fahrenheit . Grease a baking sheet lightly. 5 minutes over high heat, until a cast iron pan is blazing hot. mix the paprika, salt, cayenne pepper, cumin, thyme, white pepper, and onion powder in a mixing bowl. Cook the chicken breasts on all sides with cooking spray, then evenly cover them with the spice mixture.

Cook for 1 minute in the heated pan with the chicken. Cook for 1 minute on the opposite side. Place the breasts on the baking sheet that has been prepared. Bake for 5 minutes in a preheated oven until the center is no longer pink and the juices flow clear.

Nutrition

Per Serving: 135 calories; protein 24.7g; carbohydrates 0.9g; fat 3g; cholesterol 67.2mg; sodium 204.7mg. Full Nutrition

96. THYME-ROASTED TURKEY BREAST

Prep:10 MIN

Total:2 HR 25 MIN

Ingredients

- 1bone-in whole turkey breast (4 1/4 to 5 lb), thawed if frozen
- 1/2cup ofapple juice or dry white wine
- 2tbsp chopped fresh or 1 1/2 tsp dried thyme leaves
- 1tsp paprika
- 1/2tsp salt
- 2cloves garlic, finely chopped

Instructions

While you're cooking, be sure your screen doesn't go dark.

Preheat the oven to 325 degrees Fahrenheit. Place the turkey breast, skin side up, on a rack in a big shallow roasting pan.In the deepest tissue of the chest, insert an oven-safe meat thermometer, but without touching the bone.

Roast for 30 minutes, uncovered.

mix the remaining ingredients in a small bowl. One-third of the apple juice mixture should be brushed over the turkey.

Roast for another 1 hour to 1 hour 30 minutes, brushing with apple juice mixture every 30 minutes, or until thermometer reads 165°F. Cover with foil and let aside for 15 minutes to make carving easier.

97. ALFREDO CHICKEN WINGS

Prep:10 mins

Cook:1 hr

Total:1 hr 10 mins

Ingredients

- 3 pounds chicken wings
- 1 tbspseasoned salt
- ¼ cup ofLAND O LAKES® Salted Butter
- 1 cup ofheavy cream
- 1 tbspminced garlic
- 1 ¼ cups of grated Parmesan cheese

Instructions

Warm the oven to 375 degrees Fahrenheit. A big rimmed baking sheet should be greased. Place the wings on the baking sheet that has been prepared. Season the wings with seasoned salt and toss to coat evenly. Arrange all of the items in a single layer.Roast for 1 hour in a preheated oven until crisp and cooked through.

Turn on the oven broiler and continue crisping the wings on both sides, about 1 minute each side.

In a small saucepan, melt the butter over low heat. Stir in the cream and garlic until tiny bubbles appear. Stir in the shredded cheese before everything is thoroughly mixd. Turn off the heat in the pan.

Serve the wings with Alfredo sauce.

Note:
Method: Place frozen wings in an electric pressure cooker with a cup ofwater and cook on high pressure for 12 minutes. (When the skins have shrunk, the wings are ready to eat.) Preheat the oven to broil, then season the wings on the pan. Broil until crispy on one side, then flip, season, and broil until crispy on the other. In half the time, you can go from frozen to cooked!!

Nutrition
Per Serving: 668 calories; protein 34g; carbohydrates 4.1g; fat 57.3g; cholesterol 206mg; sodium 1280.3mg.

98. CHICKEN DRUMSTICKS

prep time: 5 MINUTES

cook time: 45 MINUTES

total time: 50 MINUTES

Ingredients

- 2 pounds chicken drumsticks
- 2 tbsp avocado oil
- 1 tsp paprika
- 1 tsp garlic powder
- 1 tsp onion powder
- 1 tsp chopped parsley
- ½ tsp salt
- ½ tsp cracked pepper

Instructions

Preheat the oven to 425 degrees Fahrenheit. Using nonstick spray, coat a baking sheet.
Seal a big zip top bag with all of the ingredients. To coat the chicken in spice, smush it about in the bag.
Place the chicken on the baking pan and bake for 40-45 minutes, or until it reaches 165 degrees on a thermometer.
Serve right away.

Nutrition

Calories323,Total Fat18g,Saturated Fat4g,Trans Fat0g,Unsaturated

Fat12g,Cholesterol192mg,Sodium325mg,Carbohydrates1g,Net Carbohydrates1g,Fiber0g,Sugar0g,Protein37g.

99. TURKEY MEATBALLS

PREP TIME:15 mins

COOK TIME:20 mins

Ingredients

- 2 pounds ground turkey 93% lean
- 1 cup ofbread crumbs or panko or rolled oats
- 2/3 cup ofonion minced
- 1/2 cup offresh parsley minced
- 2 large eggs
- 3 cloves garlic minced
- 2 tsp Worcestershire sauce
- 1/2 tsp dried basil
- 1/2 tsp dried oregano
- Salt and freshly ground black pepper
- 1/4 cup ofolive oil

Instructions

mix ground turkey, bread crumbs, onion, parsley, eggs, garlic, Worcestershire sauce, basil, oregano, 1 tsp salt, and 12 tsp pepper in a large mixing bowl.

Mix thoroughly with a sturdy spatula or your hands (latex gloves are recommended). Make 1-inch balls out of the mixture (you should have around 48 total).

To bake the meatballs, follow these steps:
Preheat the oven to 400 degrees Fahrenheit. To make cleaning easier, line a rimmed baking sheet with foil. Spray a wire rack with nonstick making spray and place it on the baking sheet.

Place meatballs on a rack, spray with oil, and bake for 15 to 20 minutes, or until browned and crispy on the edges (an internal thermometer should read 165 degrees for 15 seconds).
Fry the meatballs as follows:
In a big skillet, warm the oil over medium-high heat. Fry the meatballs in batches before they are golden brown on both sides and cooked through, about 5 to 7 minutes each batch (an internal thermometer should read 165 degrees for 15 seconds). If the skillet appears to be dry between batches, add additional oil.
To freeze the meatballs, follow these steps:
Arrange on a roasting sheet in a single layer, not touching. Freeze for 1 hour or before firm, then transfer to a freezer-safe container and keep for up to 1 month.

Nutrition

Calories: 306kcal,Carbohydrates: 14g,Protein: 35g,Fat: 12g

Saturated Fat: 2g,Trans Fat: 1g,Cholesterol: 124mg,Sodium: 220mg,Potassium: 501mg,Fiber: 1g,Sugar: 2g,Vitamin A: 475IU,Vitamin C: 7mg,Calcium: 58mg,Iron: 3mg.

100. STEAK SALAD

Prep Time: 35 mins

Cook Time: 10 mins

Total Time: 45 mins

Ingredients

- ¼ cup of balsamic vinegar
- 2 tsp dijon mustard
- 1 tsp mayonnaise, optional
- ½ tsp kosher salt
- ¼ tsp black pepper
- ½ cup of extra-virgin vegetable oil

Steak Salad

- 1 pound straightening iron steaks or skirt steak
- kosher sodium chloride, for seasoning
- black pepper, for seasoning
- 2 tbsp olive oil
- 4 cups of arugula, 1-inch pieces
- 4 cups of romaine lettuce
- 2 cups of radicchio, 1-inch pieces
- 1 cup of cherry tomatoes, cut in half
- ½ cup of thinly sliced cucumber
- ¼ cup of thinly sliced radish
- ¼ cup of diced red onion
- 1 medium avocado, sliced or diced
- ¼ cup of feta cheese

Instructions

Whisk together the vinegar, mustard, mayonnaise, salt, and pepper in a medium mixing basin.

Slowly trickle in the olive oil, whisking constantly, until the dressing has thickened and emulsified.

Using paper towels, dry the steak's surface.

Season with salt and pepper on both sides.

Until a big cast-iron skillet is hot, heat it over high fire. Once the oil is heated, add the steak and firmly press it into the pan. Cook for 4 minutes, or until the surface is browned.

Cook for another 3 to 5 minutes, or until the steak achieves an internal temperature of 120 to 125°F (49 to 52°C) for medium-rare.

Place the steak on a chopping board and let aside for 10 minutes to rest. Cut the meat into 14-inch thick slices against the grain. If you want to cook it smaller, do so.

 mix the arugula, romaine, and radicchio in a large serving bowl.

The salad is topped with tomatoes, cucumber, radish, onion, beef, avocado, and feta cheese.

Serve with a balsamic vinaigrette on top of the steak salad.

101. SESAME BEEF STIR FRY

PREP:15 MINS

COOK:12 MINS

MARINATING TIME:15 MINS

TOTAL:27 MINS

INGREDIENTS
BEEF MARINADE

- 2 tsp minced garlic
- 1 Tbsp grated fresh ginger
- 2 Tbsp reduced sodium soy sauce
- 1 Tbsp rice vinegar
- 1 Tbsp sesame oil
- 1 Tbsp sesame seeds
- 1/2 tsp Chinese 5 spice
- 1/4 tsp black pepper

STIR FRY

- 1 lb flank steak, thinly sliced
- 1 cups ofnow peas, sliced in half across
- 1/2 cups ofliced carrots
- 8 green onions, sliced
- 1/4 cup ofbeef broth
- 2 Tbsp reduced sodium soy sauce
- 1-2 Tbsp honey or light brown sugar
- 1 Tbsp rice vinegar

- 1/2 Tbsp minced garlic
- 2 tsp sesame oil
- 1 tsp grated fresh ginger
- 1 tsp cornstarch
- 1/2 tsp red pepper flakes
- 2 Tbsp vegetable oil (for cooking)

INSTRUCTIONS

In a mixing bowl, mix the marinate ingredients and add the flank steak. Allow 15 minutes for preparation.

In a large pan, heat 1 tbspvegetable oil over MED HIGH heat. Remove the extra marinade from the steak and fry it in a single layer for 2-3 minutes, stirring halfway through to ensure even cooking. Based on the size of your pan, you may need to do this in batches. Arrange the meat on a serving dish.

Heat the remaining 1 tbspvegetable oil, then add the peas, carrots, and green onion and simmer for 2-3 minutes, turning often.

Broth, soy sauce, honey/brown sugar, rice vinegar, garlic, sesame oil, fresh ginger, cornstarch, and red pepper flakes should all be whisked together. Stir the meat and sauce together in the skillet. The sauce will thicken over time.

If using, add cooked ramen noodles and serve!

102. BEEF FILLET STEAKS WITH PEPPER THYME SAUCE

EADY IN: 30mins

INGREDIENTS

- 1tbspolive oil
- 4steak fillets
- 1celery rib, finely chopped
- 2garlic cloves, crushed
- 1brown onion, chopped finely
- 1/2cup ofdry white wine
- 1tsp beef stock granules
- 300ml double cream
- 1tsp ground mixed peppercorns (or more)
- 1tbspfresh thyme leave

DIRECTIONS

In a big frying pan, heat half the oil and cook the meat on both sides until done to your liking. To keep warm, transfer to a heated oven.

If you have big steaks like mine, you won't be able to cook them to medium rare on the stove without scorching the outside, so you'll need to finish them in the oven for around 15 minutes at a higher heat level.

In the same pan, warm the remaining oil, then add the celery, onion, and garlic and cook, turning occasionally, until the veggies are softened.

Stir in the wine until the liquid has been reduced by half, then add the cream, peppercorns, and stock and bring to a boil. Reduce warm to low and make, uncovered, for approximately 5 minutes, or until sauce thickens slightly. Add the thyme leaves and serve over the meat right away.

Serve with your favorite vegetables and potatoes. I served mine with celeriac mash and a carrot casserole as a side.

103. CRANBERRY MEATBALLS

Total Time

Prep: 20 min.

Bake: 20 min.

Ingredients

- 2 large eggs, lightly beaten
- 1 cup ofcornflake crumbs
- 1/3 cup ofketchup
- 2 tbsp dried minced onion
- 2 tbsp soy sauce
- 1 tbspdried parsley flakes
- 1/2 tsp salt
- 1/4 tsp pepper
- 2 pounds ground pork

SAUCE:

- 1 can (14 ounces) jellied cranberry sauce
- 1 cup ofketchup
- 3 tbsp brown sugar
- 1 tbsplemon juice

Directions

Preheat the oven to 350 degrees Fahrenheit.Blend the first eight items in a bowl. Mix in the pork lightly but thoroughly. Form meatballs that are 1 inch in diameter. In a 15x10x1-in. pan, place on a greased rack. Cook for 20-25 minutes, or until a thermometer reaches 160°. Meatballs should be drained on paper towels.

Cook and whisk the sauce ingredients in a large pan over medium heat until well mixd. Add the meatballs and cook thoroughly.

Nutrition

1 meatball: 58 calories, 2g fat (1g saturated fat), 16mg cholesterol, 142mg sodium, 6g carbohydrate (4g sugars, 0 fiber), 3g protein.

104. BEEF FILLET STEAKS WITH PEPPER THYME SAUCE

READY IN: 30mins

SERVES: 4

INGREDIENTS

- 1 tbsp olive oil
- 4 steak fillets
- 1 celery rib, finely chopped
- 2 garlic cloves, crushed
- 1 brown onion, chopped finely
- 1/2 cup of dry white wine
- 1 tsp beef stock granules
- 300 ml double cream
- 1 tsp ground mixed peppercorns (or more)
- 1 tbsp fresh thyme leave

DIRECTIONS

In a big frying pan, heat half the oil and cook the meat on both sides until done to your liking. To keep warm, transfer to a heated oven.

If you have big steaks like mine, you won't be able to cook them to medium rare on the stove without scorching the outside, so you'll need to finish them in the oven for around 15 minutes at a higher heat level.

In the same pan, warm the remaining oil, then add the celery, onion, and garlic and cook, turning occasionally, until the veggies are softened.

Stir in the wine until the liquid has been reduced by half, then add the cream, peppercorns, and stock and bring to a boil. Reduce warm to low and cook, uncovered, for approximately 5 minutes, or until sauce thickens slightly. Add the thyme leaves and serve over the meat right away.

Serve with your favorite vegetables and potatoes. I served mine with celeriac mash and a carrot casserole as a side.

NUTRITION INFO

Serving Size: 1 (149) g

Servings Per Recipe: 4

AMT. PER SERVING:Calories: 333.9,Calories from Fat 285 g,Total Fat 31.7 g,Saturated Fat 18.1 g,Cholesterol 104.8 mg,Sodium 39.7 mg,Total Carbohydrate 6.6 g,Dietary Fiber 0.7 g,Sugars 1.7 g,Protein 2 g.

105. HONEY GARLIC PORK CHOPS

PREP:10 MINS

COOK:12 MINS

TOTAL:22 MINS

INGREDIENTS

- 4 pork chops bone in or out
- Salt and pepper, to season
- 1 tsp garlic powder
- 2 tbsp olive oil
- 1 tbsp unsalted butter
- 6 cloves garlic, minced
- 1/4 cup of honey
- 1/4 cup of water
- 2 tbsp rice wine vinegar

INSTRUCTIONS

warm the broiler in the oven to medium-high. Just before cooking, season the chops with salt, pepper, and garlic powder.

In a pan or skillet, heat the oil over medium high heat until it is hot. Chops should be seared on all sides until golden brown and cooked thoroughly (about 4-5 minutes each side). Place on a platter and put away.

Reduce to a medium heat setting. In the same pan, melt butter, scraping away any browned pieces from the bottom. Garlic should be sautéed until aromatic (about 30 seconds). mix the honey, water, and vinegar in a mixing bowl. Increase the heat to medium-high and simmer, stirring periodically, until the sauce has reduced and thickened somewhat (approximately 3-4 minutes).

Return the pork to the pan, baste with sauce, and broil/grill for 1-2 minutes, or until the edges are slightly browned.

Enjoy with parsley-garnished vegetables, rice, pasta, or a salad.

NOTES

Preheat oven to 390°F | 200°C for baked pork chops.

Sear seasoned chops for 2 minutes each side in a hot oven-proof pan or skillet over medium-high heat to crisp them up.

Remove the chops and prepare the sauce as directed in the recipe (Step 3).

Baste with sauce and bake for about 10-15 minutes, or until desired doneness is achieved.

To obtain those caramelized edges, broil/grill for 2 minutes.

NUTRITION

Calories: 332kcal | Carbohydrates: 15g | Protein: 29g | Fat: 12g | Saturated Fat: 5g | Cholesterol: 104mg | Sodium: 68mg | Potassium: 337mg | Sugar: 14g | Vitamin A: 175IU | Vitamin C: 1.4mg | Calcium: 18mg | Iron: 0.8mg

106. HAM WITH ORANGE-APRICOT SAUCE

Prep: 10 min.

Bake: 1-1/2 hours

Ingredients

- 1 bone-in fully made spiral-sliced ham
- 1 cup ofthawed orange juice concentrate
- 1 cups ofugar
- 1 cup ofdried apricots, chopped
- 1/2 cup ofwater
- 1/2 cup ofdried cranberries
- 3 tbsp dried currants

Directions

In a small roasting pan, place the ham on a rack. Cover and bake for 2 1/2 to 3 hours at 325°F, or until a thermometer registers 140°F.

 mix the juice concentrate, sugar, apricots, water, cranberries, and currants in a large saucepan. Bring the water to a boil. Reduce warm to low and make, uncovered, for 3-5 minutes, or until sauce has thickened somewhat. Serve with ham on the side.

Nutrition

1 each: 384 calories, 5g fat , 47mg cholesterol, 1906mg sodium, 47g carbohydrate, 39g protein.

107. SAUSAGE, PEPPERS, AND ONIONS

, PREP TIME:10 mins

COOK TIME:40 mins

TOTAL TIME:50 mins

Ingredients

- 4 Italian sausage links (sweet, hot, or a couple of each)
- 2 tbsp extra virgin olive oil
- 1green bell pepper, sliced into 3 inch strips
- 1 red bell pepper, sliced into 3 inch strips
- 1 bell pepper of another color (yellow or orange or purple), sliced into 3-inch strips
- 4 garlic cloves, sliced into slivers
- 1 large yellow onion, sliced into 1/4-inch half-moons
- 1 (15-ounce) can crushed tomatoes
- 1 tbspdried oregano
- 1/2 cup ofMarsala or red wine, optional
- 1/2 tsp red pepper flakes, optional
- Salt as need

Directions

Brown the sausages: In a large pan with a cover, heat the olive oil over medium heat. Add the sausages to the heated oil and brown them slowly.

Reduce the heat if they're sizzling and crackling too much. A gradual browning, not a sear, is desired. Cook for a few minutes, turning them occasionally to ensure even browning. When the sausage have brown, take them from the pan and set them aside.

the Italian sausages should be browned

Sauté the onions, peppers, and garlic in the following order:

Add the onions and peppers and turn the heat up to high. Toss them in the pan to coat them with oil and sear them as best you can, stirring occasionally.

Sprinkle salt over the onions and peppers once they've softened. Once the onions and peppers have blackened from a thorough sear, add the garlic and simmer for another minute.

Optional: deglaze pan with wine

If used, pour in the Marsala or red wine. To release all the browned and blackened pieces, scrape the bottom of the pan with a metal spatula or wooden spoon. Allow the wine to reduce by half.

All of the components should be simmered together:

 mix the tomatoes, oregano, and red pepper flakes (if using) in a large mixing bowl. Return the sausages to the pan. Bring to a low boil, then reduce to a low heat. Reduce the heat to a low setting.

Cover and cook for 20 minutes, or until the peppers are soft and the sausages are cooked through.

108. CHOCOLATE CHIP COOKIE RECIPE

PREP TIME:10 mins

COOK TIME:8 mins

TOTAL TIME:30 mins

EQUIPMENT

- measuring spoons
- measuring cups of
- KitchenAid Mixer
- spatula
- baking sheet

INGREDIENTS

- 1 cups ofalted butter softened
- 1 cup ofwhite (granulated) sugar
- 1 cup oflight brown sugar packed
- 2 tsp pure vanilla extract
- 2 large eggs
- 3 cups of all-purpose flour
- 1 tsp baking soda
- ½ tsp baking powder
- 1 tsp sea salt
- 2 cups of chocolate chips (or chunks, or chopped chocolate)

INSTRUCTIONS

Preheat the oven to 375 degrees Fahrenheit. Set aside a baking tray lined with parchment paper.

mix flour, baking soda, salt, and baking powder in a separate basin. Eliminate from the equation.

Cream the butter and sugars together until smooth.

Using an electric blender, beat in the eggs and lemon zest until frothy.

Blend in the dry ingredients before everything is well mixed.

Mix in a 12 oz container of chocolate chips well.

Roll 2-3 TBS of dough into balls at a time (depending on how big you prefer your cookies) and set them equally spread on the prepared cookie sheets. (Alternatively, make your cookies with a tiny cookie scoop.)

warm the oven to 350°F and roast for 8-10 minutes. Pull them when they are just beginning to turn brown.

Allow them to cool for 2 minutes on the baking sheet before transferring to a cooling rack.

NUTRITION

Serving: 1cookie (using 3 TBS dough)

Calories: 183kcal,Carbohydrates: 26g,Protein: 2g,Fat: 8g,Saturated Fat: 5g,Cholesterol: 27mg,Sodium: 153mg,Potassium: 31mg,Fiber: 1g,Sugar: 18g,Vitamin A: 197IU,Vitamin C: 1mg,Calcium: 24mg,Iron: 1mg

109. GARLIC AND ROSEMARY GRILLED LAMB CHOPS

Prep Time:15 minutes

Cook Time:10 minutes

Total Time:25 minutes

Ingredients

- 2 pounds lamb loin
- 4 cloves garlic minced
- 1 tbspfresh rosemary chopped
- 1 1/4 tsp kosher salt
- 1/2 tsp ground black pepper
- zest of 1 lemon
- 1/4 cup ofolive oil

Instructions

In a measuring cup, mix the garlic, rosemary, salt, pepper, lemon zest, and olive oil.

Flip the lamb chunks over the mixture to coat them well. Refrigerate the chops for as little as 1 hour or as long as overnight, covered.

Grill the lamb chops for 7-10 minutes over medium heat, or until they reach an internal temperature of 135 degrees F.

Allow cooked lamb chops to rest on a platter covered with aluminum foil for 5 minutes before serving.

110. HAM WITH ORANGE-APRICOT SAUCE

Total Time Prep: 10 min. Bake: 1-1/2 hours

Makes:15 servings (2-1/4 cups of sauce)

Ingredients

- 1 bone-in fully cooked spiral-sliced ham
- 1 cup ofthawed orange juice concentrate
- 1 cups ofugar
- 1 cup ofdried apricots, chopped
- 1/2 cup ofwater
- 1/2 cup ofdried cranberries
- 3 tbsp dried currants

Directions

In a small roasting pan, place the ham on a rack. Cover and bake for 2 1/2 to 3 hours at 325°F, or until a thermometer registers 140°F.

 mix the juice concentrate, sugar, apricots, water, cranberries, and currants in a large saucepan. Bring the water to a boil. Reduce warm to low and make, uncovered, for 3-5 minutes, or until sauce has thickened somewhat. Serve with ham on the side.

Nutrition Facts

1 each: 384 calories, 5g fat , 47mg cholesterol, 1906mg sodium, 47g carbohydrate, 39g protein.

CONCLISION

Printed in the USA
CPSIA information can be obtained
at www.ICGtesting.com
LVHW050816301124
798007LV00011B/638